Dear Jane,

Thank you a_
of our retreat. It's magical re
the universe brings people together.

ONE YOGA

I hope you find this simple
practice guide helpful. All answers
can be found through the earnest
desire to learn and dedication to
practice. Your
           Own
           Great
           Awareness.
                    Wishing you light,
                    love + blessings

Susan
Sm__

One-Yoga Publication
Wilmington, Delaware 19807

Credits:
Cover Photography by Eric Trockenbrot
Cover Design by David Teague, Inteloquence, LLC
Content Photography by Barbara Grabher
Author's Photograph by Eric Trockenbrot

Contents

Acknowledgments

I would like to thank all of the teachers who influence me and help me as I deepen my own yoga practice. There is something to be learned from every person you meet. Family and friends lovingly contributed time, direction and support for this endeavor.

My special thanks go to:

- my husband, Robbie, who has always believed that I could do whatever I set my mind to. Your support, understanding and love made this possible;
- my sons, Gregory and Douglas, who sacrificed Mommy time so that I could think, work and practice;
- my mom and dad, Janet and Tim, who allowed me to fly as a child—instilling in me confidence and determination, with the gift of Christian principles;
- my sister-in-law Priscilla—I would not have been able to tackle this project without your editorial expertise. You jumped in willingly and knowingly. Thank you for your commitment;
- Barbara Grabher who's kindness, generosity and excellent professional photography effortlessly captured the essence of all the asanas;
- Kerry Orr, my friend. You joyfully and graciously offered your time and yoga expertise guiding me through the photo shoot;
- Debbie Cutler, who gave me the room for growth and supported my developmental path. Her encouragement and vision is inspiring.
- my dear friend Theresa Fackler, who pushed me to go higher, look further and believe that I can. Her input and suggestions kept me on track.
- all my friends and family members who listened to me endlessly talk about yoga.

I am most grateful and blessed for all who have participated in my classes, workshops and trainings. Each and every one of you has taught me something that I carry in my heart. For everyone that God has put in my path, I am forever thankful.

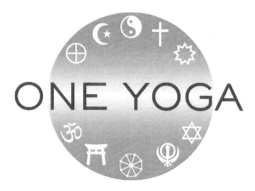

Mission Statement

To teach yoga to everyone who has the desire to learn guiding each practice with love and intuition. To use my experiences and knowledge to help practitioners on their journey by being fully present and discovering the physical, mental, emotional and spiritual needs of each person. And, through this discovery and understanding, aid in the restoration of balance, well-being and peace.

Introduction

Welcome to **"The Power of Yoga"**!

This book is for individuals interested in learning power flow yoga. This style of teaching is derived from my life experiences, training and practice. It is based on the belief that yoga is for everyone. There is no correct or incorrect yoga practice; only that which is appropriate for each individual utilizing safe and intuitive guidelines.

The power behind Power Flow Yoga comes from the active physical asana practice, which is designed to open the body, mind and heart to a new way of life. I was originally attracted to Power Flow Yoga because it challenged me physically. So much so, that my ego had to step aside and surrender. It is in that surrender that I realized my potential for peace, stillness and love.

"The Power of Yoga" is designed to be used as a guide for asana practice. It is through regular practice that one discovers the benefits of Power Flow Yoga. Each person undergoes self-exploration and discovery as their commitment to yoga deepens, both on and off the mat. This style of practice unfolds to each person differently. Work, belief systems and life experiences influence each practitioner. Through dedication and regular practice, individuals begin to uncover the true self that lies dormant in each of us. It is through that awakening that the asana practice flowers into something much greater. My hope is to share what I have learned to help others on their path.

Please let me clarify for those new to yoga that yoga is not a religion, although many find their spirituality and connectedness through practice. Yoga is an ancient philosophy developed thousands of years ago. Its original intention focused on maintaining a healthy mind, body and soul, with an end-point vision of connecting to the divine within each of us.

There are different pathways of yoga. They outline five different routes that can be taken on this journey of self-discovery. They are:
Jnana Yoga or the Yoga of Knowledge
Bhakti Yoga or the Yoga of Devotion
Kriya Yoga or the Yoga of Technique
Karma Yoga or the Yoga of Service
Raja Yoga known as Royal Yoga or Integral Path Yoga, which combines all four.

There are many different styles or various techniques of practice within the pathways of yoga. Exploration of these varying styles and methods is valuable. One-Yoga's Power Flow format is one of these styles. It utilizes a practical, straight forward approach that is based on universal truths. For the purpose of this book we'll concentrate on five basic practice components that are the foundation of One-Yoga's Power Flow Yoga. They are:

1. Breath (Pranayama)
2. Pose (Asana)
3. Gaze (Drishti)
4. Flow (Vinyasa)
5. Relaxation and Meditation (Dhyana)

Throughout my experience, I have learned that most people's physical bodies are tight, their minds are busy and their spirit is buried. One-Yoga uses a basic class structure to allow for these opportunities. Our practice offers each student the time to gradually assess and progress through the practice enabling the bodies to open, the minds to settle and the spirit to breathe. Our journey begins with the physical practice of yoga or better known as asana practice. It is instrumental in unlocking the emotional and spiritual doorways to a higher level of consciousness. One-Yoga's basic class structure includes the following:

- Assessment Series
- Warm-Up Series (traditional Sun Salutations)
- Primary Standing Flow
- Secondary Standing Flow
- Balancing Asanas
- Back-Bending Series
- Core Work
- Hip-Opening Series
- Closing Series

The goal of this book is two-fold: introduce Power Flow Yoga to those exploring this style of practice; and serve as reference for those cultivating their own home practice. The methodology is well-rounded, cultivating muscular strength and stamina, while increasing joint range of motion and overall flexibility as part of a detoxifying physical practice that reduces stress and increases serenity. It is important to remember to honor yourself.

People begin practicing yoga for a variety of reasons: To lose weight, tone muscles, increase flexibility, heal back, neck or shoulder issues, improve a golf game, increase ability to focus, reduce stress, and compliment other fitness activities. These are just a few and are all wonderful reasons to begin a yoga regime. However, the reason people return over and over to yoga practice is because it enables them to become more fully present in their daily lives. Any reason or motivation for beginning is great. It's your starting point.

We live in a world of technology and competition. Our lives have become increasingly crazy. Our "to-do-lists" never end. Our society rewards multi-tasking and fosters the ability to do more in less time. But, what have we really created? When we are talking with a neighbor, co-worker, spouse or child, are we really listening? Or are we formulating our next activity or action that needs to be taken based on that endless chatter that rattles off in our heads. So let your starting point – be just that, a beginning without expectation or judgment. Permit yourself the opportunity to do as much or as little of this practice as you can. Just do it, and keep doing it. I always say the magic number is five. You need to consistently practice for five days in a row before you begin to feel the mental, physical and soulful benefits. If you can take a class from a qualified competent instructor, all the better. It will contribute and complement your own practice. It's just you and your mat.

Everyone who practices yoga comes with some baggage. It may be mental or emotional stress, physical limitations or preconceived notions. That's O.K., you've taken the first step. Whenever you go on vacation, you have to unpack the luggage before the vacation begins. Once you've emptied the suitcase, the fun starts. It's the same way in yoga. Be mindful. Be kind to yourself. Be patient. It takes time. Listen with intuition. Feeling uncomfortable is perfectly fine, but pain should be avoided. Meeting your edge and facing fears is a healthy form of growth. Allowing your ego to push you so far that you fall off the cliff blocks advancement and self-realization. Hopefully the journey will enlighten your life, and enable you to live each moment fully present.

Five Basic Practice Components

The **Breath of Life** (**pranayama**) is the most important of the five components, for without breath there is no life. There are many types of pranayama or breathing techniques, but for our purposes, we will focus on one—Ujjayi (victorious) breath. In its most basic form, Ujjayi breath engages a series of bandhas. The three we will review are Mulabandha, Uddiyana, and Jalandhara Bandha. The bandhas are doorways to energy flow (prana) within the body. They are often referred to as locks. Mulabandha means root and is located at the base of the spine. Uddiyana means flying up or soaring and is used to refer to the core or abdominal lock. The Jalandhara Bandha or water pipe lock refers to a chin lock that is used to retain and regulate prana.

> "Breathing may be considered the most important of all the functions of the body, for, indeed, all the other functions depend upon it."—*Ramacharaka: Hindu-Yogi Science of Breath*

> "Pranayama is what heart is to the human body."—B.K. Iyengar: *Light on the Yoga Sutras of Patanjali*

Poses (**asanas**) are specific body positions that have physical, mental, neurological, and emotional benefits. When most newcomers refer to "yoga," they are often referring to the physical practice of asana. Although asana is a key ingredient, yoga is much more than the physical practice of bodily positions.

> Wikipedia Encyclopedia gives us the following definitions: Asana is Sanskrit for "seat." The plural is used to describe yoga postures; "seat" in this context refers not only to the physical position of the body, but to the position of the spirit in relation to divinity. This idea is often referred to as the "one seat" by yogis and Buddhists alike.

> Modern usage of the word "asana" in reference to the practice of yoga generally intends the former definition of a physical posture or pose. In the *Yoga Sutra*, Patanjali describes "asana" as sitting meditation, where meditation is the path to self-realization. "Asana," therefore, means both simple postures and a path to unity of spirit.

Although "asana" originally referred to sitting meditation, its scope has evolved over centuries to cover a great variety of body postures. These postures have their roots in devotion and/or health, but ultimately all are intended to lead back to the possibility of sitting more comfortably in meditation.

Gaze (drishti) is a point of focus where your eyes come to rest. In asana and meditation practice there is a suggested focal point or drishti to help maintain stillness and presence. When eyes settle on a drishti, concentration is improved, pranayama slows, and the body begins to stabilize. Drishti is also used to help maintain appropriate alignment especially of the spine.

A drishti (view or gaze) is a specific focal point that is employed during meditation or while holding a yoga posture. The ancient yogis discovered that where our gaze is directed, our attention naturally follows, and that the quality of our gazing is directly reflected in the quality of our mental thoughts. When the gaze is fixed on a single point the mind is diminished from being stimulated by all other external objects. And when the gaze is fixed on a single point within the body, our awareness draws inwards and the mind remains undisturbed by external stimuli. Thus, the use of a drishti allows the mind to focus and move into a deep state of concentration. And the constant application of drishti develops ekagraha, single-pointed focus, an essential yogic technique used to still the mind. "Focusing on a Drishti"—*Yoga Basics*

Flow describes **vinyasa**, a sequence of linked poses. Sun salutations are an example of vinyasa. Linking one pose to the next connected with breath is vinyasa flow yoga. In this training, transitions are a form of flow or vinyasa. Typically, inhalations are used in connection with the opening of the body and exposing the heart center. Exhalations are linked with movements that close the body or compress the belly—they are stabilizing and grounding.

The word vinyasa can be broken down into its Sanskrit roots to assist us in finding its meaning. *Nyasa* means "to place" and *vi* means "in a special way." One common interpretation of vinyasa then is a breath-synchronized movement; breath and movement are seamlessly united in such a way that each action encourages the other. For each movement, there is a corresponding breath.

According to the ashtanga tradition, the purpose of
linking the breath with movement (vinyasa) is internal
cleansing. Vinyasa generates the subtle, internal heat
of transformation and stokes agni fire. Agni is the
digestive fire used not only to digest physical food but
also experiences and sensations. If our fire is strong,
we can better adapt to life's challenges. *The Many
Nuances of Vinyasa*—Lori Gaspar

Relaxation and **meditation** can be achieved in a variety of formats. **Dhyana
(meditation)** is the connection obtained through focused attention. As we
deliberately direct our thoughts and awareness to a single point, we are able to
release and detach from the multi-tasking noisy mind. As the mind relinquishes
control, intimacy with stillness flourishes. This relationship is Dhyana: a step or
path to Samadhi—a state of joy, bliss and peace.

There are countless types of meditation, and the exploration of these various
techniques is an enlightening experience. Although you may experience
moments or periods of meditative states throughout the practice, we will reserve
the relaxation/meditation for the conclusion of our practice. The quietening of
our mind begins during savasana and is the fruit of our labor.

Emerson wrote, "To the illumined mind, the whole
world sparkles with light." So how do we illuminate
our minds to see the world as a child sees it? How do
we let go of all of the mental baggage we carry
around with us? Yoga and meditation are doorways
to discover that mind again—a mind that knows
stillness and relief, a mind that experiences peace
and rediscovers a sense of wonder at simply being
alive.

Dhyana is our ability to sustain attention and focus without distraction in the
journey to samadhi (union/bringing into harmony) the ultimate intention of
meditation. Through this practice we become completely absorbed and
connected to the divine within. This is the joyful bliss and fulfillment of life as we
become one with all.

Assessment Series

One-Yoga applies the five basic principles of yoga throughout the class, starting with Assessment. The Assessment begins with breath, and continues with 3 or 4 poses that allow you to determine your current physical, mental, and emotional well-being at the moment.

Start in Child's Pose. Begin to tune into your breath. The Ujjayi breath requires awareness and engagement of the bandhas or also known as locks. All breathing for Ujjayi is maintained through the nose and nasal passageways. Pranayama or the "Breath of Life" is the most important component of yoga, for without breath there is no life. So, let's take a few moments and work through understanding how to initiate and maintain the Ujjayi breath. Let's begin with Mulabandha. The root lock or Mulabandha is located at the base of your spine, the pelvic floor. To initiate Mulabandha an internal lift of the pelvic floor is needed. The perineum is an area located between the anus and genitalia. Bring your focus to the perineum or pelvic floor, and begin to inwardly lift the internal root muscles. Maintain that engagement or lock throughout inhalation and exhalation to tap into Mulabandha. Uddiyana Bandha is a bit easier to master. As you muscularly draw the naval into the spine restricting the diaphragmatic descent, you begin to feel the expansive benefits of the belly lock or Uddiyana Bandha. Continue to maintain nice even inhalations and exhalations. Uddiyana Bandha forces the diaphragm upward into the body, requiring the ribcage and lungs to expand front to back and side to side. The final lock used in the Ujjayi breath is Jalandhara Bandha or also known as the water pipe or chin lock. This lock creates an audible sound similar to wind moving though trees. It requires a partial restriction of the glottis. The glottis is generally located at the base of the throat between the collar bones. As you begin to partially close off the glottis and inhale, you will hear the raspy noise associated with the Ujjayi Pranayama. Maintain the partial constriction of the glottis as you exhale through the nose. As you practice Jalandhara Bandha, you will feel the air passing the nasal passages and throat. Ujjayi Breath is attained through attention to all three bandhas throughout even and rhythmical inhalations and exhalations.

The Ujjayi (victorious) breath is key to this practice because of the physiological effects it induces. Most notably the Ujjayi breath ignites the parasympathetic nervous system which induces a state of calm, and prevents the body from going into the "fight or flight" mode. Complete 5 to 10 breath cycles, dropping all thoughts and becoming present in the moment. Take your time. Allow yourself the opportunity to tap into the breath and body. Honor yourself and move within your own limitations. Modify the poses if need be. Don't go so deep, feel free to move into a less challenging version of the pose and please leave the ego at the door. There are numerous reasons why a particular asana is difficult – remember this can be attributed to physical disabilities, injuries or limitations, mental blocks, personal struggles, or spiritual issues. Be mindful. Be empathetic. Be loving.

Pose 1: Child's Pose (Balasana)

This is an active Child's Pose. Knees are spread the width of the mat--big toes touching, tops of the feet relaxing into the earth. Fold forward and allow the chest to sink between the legs, as the arms reach forward, palms pressed into the floor. Buttocks are sitting back on the heels as the upper body is extended, creating length. Drishti: the floor or tip of nose.

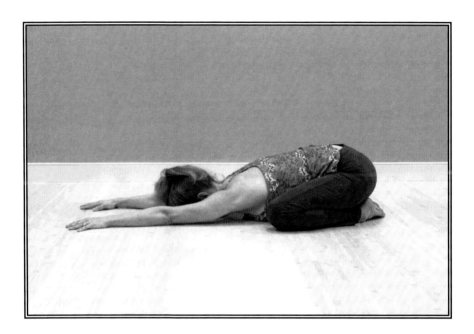

HOLD FOR 5 BREATHS

Transition: Curl toes under and press back to **Pose 2, Downward Facing Dog**

Pose 2: Downward Facing Dog
(Adho Mukha Svanasana)

Stretch and shift side to side – move around in the first **Downward Facing Dog** and work out the kinks.

This pose looks like an upside down V--arms are shoulder distance apart, legs are hip distance width. Allow the chest to press toward the thighs. Press through the quadriceps and eventually work so that the heels are down and there is equal weight distribution between the four points touching the earth. Tilt the sitting bones to the heavens and engage through the abdominals. Drishti: a spot on the floor between the feet or big toes.

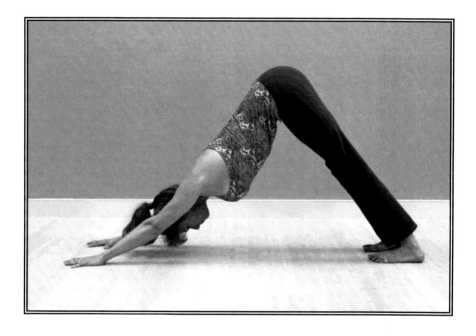

HOLD FOR 5 BREATHS

Transition: Slowly walk the feet, heel to toe, and come up into **Ragdoll**.

Pose 3: Ragdoll (Uttanasana)

Feet are separated hip distance apart. Soften the knees and hang upside down, allowing blood to enter the head and relaxing through the entire spine. Engage the quadriceps, lifting the kneecaps toward the heart to stretch and work the hamstrings. Let the arms hang heavy or clasp opposite elbows. Drop the crown of the head to the floor and gently shake the head "Yes" and "No", releasing through the neck. Drishti: belly button or base of spine.

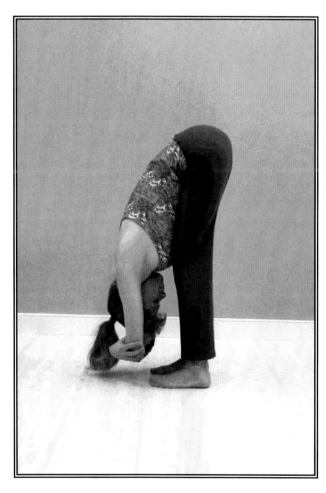

HOLD FOR 5 BREATHS

Transition: Slowly curl up one vertebra at a time, toe-heel the feet together and come into **Mountain Pose**.

Pose 4: Mountain Pose (Tadasana)

Feet are together and rooting down to the earth. Try to distribute the weight evenly on the four corners of the feet. Bring the spine into alignment, the head centered over the shoulders, shoulders over hips, hips over feet, scoop the pelvis slightly forward. Open the heart and lift through the sternum. Pull the shoulders back and release them down the spine. Drishti: a spot directly in front of the eyes or tip of nose.

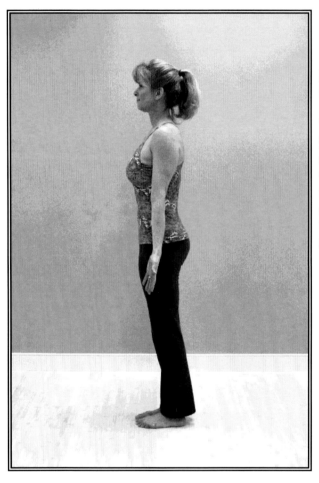

HOLD FOR 5 BREATHS

Transition: Bring hands to heart center and lift them to the sky—stretch the body upward and begin the **Warm-Up Series Sun Salutation A**.

Warm-Up Series: Sun Salutations

Sun Salutation (**Salute to the Sun**) is like a morning wake-up call. Sun Salutations are used in **One-Yoga's Power Flow Yoga**™ as a warm-up for the entire body, to enliven and invigorate the body both internally and externally. Sun Salutations use all the major muscle groups, and a breath sequence to generate internal body heat. Maintain the Ujjayi breath. It is used to complete each asana (posture) within the vinyasa (flow) of Sun Salutation A & B. Allow the breath to lead the movement and complete each pose within the vinyasa. Ujjayi breathing also helps to internalize and recirculate heat. Sun Salutation Series can change from teacher to teacher. We will study a traditional Suryanamaskar series with an additional breath and movement in the B sequence to enable practioners to get into the flow.

The **Warm-Up Series** is designed to prepare the body for development, healing and detoxification. The combination of movements and breath utilization exercise the cardiovascular system. The increased blood flow prepares muscles for our standing postures. Hold the poses for longer periods of time if needed. Listen to what your body is telling you. What is tight? What is rigid? What is jerky? Are the joint systems stacked and aligned? Chaturanga Dandasana (moving from high to low push-up position) is challenging. Please drop the knees to the floor and modify the push-up position to relieve any discomfort or strain on the shoulders / arms. In time you will gain the relevant core and leg strength to move through this asana with grace, integrity and humility.

Keep breathing and build the poses from the ground up.

Sun Salutation Series A (Surynamaskar A)

Begin in **Mountain Pose (Tadasana)**.

Inhale and extend both arms overhead, palms pressing.

Exhale and fold forward, hinging at the hips and coming through flat back to **Forward Bend (Uttanasana)**.

Inhale to **Extended Forward Bend (Urdhva Mukha Uttanasana)**, with a flat back from the base of the spine to the crown of the head.

Exhale and step or hop back to **Full Plank (Isa Dandasana)**.

Keep exhaling through **Chaturanga Dandasana**, moving from high to low push-up position.

Inhale rolling over the toes (**Yogi Toe Roll**) to **Upward Facing Dog (Urdhva Mukha Svanasana)**.

Exhale to **Downward Facing Dog (Adho Mukha Svanasana)**.

Stay in Downward Facing Dog for 3 to 5 breaths or longer if needed.

On the final exhalation, empty the lungs, and walk, hop or float forward bringing the feet up to meet the hands.

Inhale to an **Extended Forward Bend (Urdhva Mukha Uttanasana)**.

Exhale to **Forward Bend (Uttanasana)**.

Inhale, pressing through the feet, engaging the quadriceps and coming through flat back and return to **Mountain Pose (Tadasana)**.

Repeat vinyasa 2-4 times.

Sun Salutation Series A (Surynamaskar A)

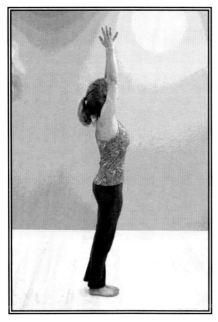

Inhale and extend both arms overhead, palms pressing.

Alignment:

- Head centered over shoulders, shoulders aligned over hips, hips stacked over feet.
- Arms reach overhead while shoulder blades release down the spine.
- Root down evenly through the four corners of the feet.
- Pelvic floor facing the earth.
- Bandhas engaged.

Exhale and fold forward, hinging at the hips to **Extended Forward Bend (Urdhva Mukha Uttanasana)**.

Alignment:

- Extend through the crown of the head.
- Abdominals draw inward toward the spine maintaining a flat back.
- Lift and engage the quadriceps. Soften the knees if needed or straighten the legs if hamstring flexibility permits.
- Hands move through heart center or arms extend out to the sides to relieve pressure on the lower back.

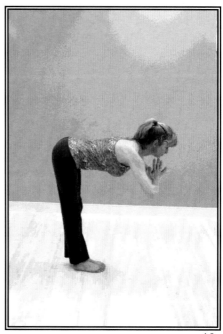

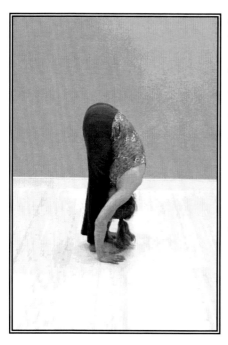

Continue to exhale and empty the lungs to **Forward Bend (Uttanasana)**.

Alignment:

- Hips aligned over heels.
- Torso draped against thighs.
- Soften through the knees as much as needed. If flexibility allows, straighten the legs and lift through the knee caps -dynamically engage the thigh muscles.
- Finger tips in line with the toes or lightly touching the floor.

Inhale to **Extended Forward Bend (Urdhva Mukha Uttanasana)**, with a flat back from the base of the spine to the crown of the head.

Alignment:

- Hips aligned over heels.
- Shoulder blades releasing back toward the midline of the body.
- Draw the belly inward.
- Thigh muscles engage and lift.
- Relax through the toes and actively involve the balls of the feet.
- Optional Modification: Rest the hands on the shins and soften the knees.

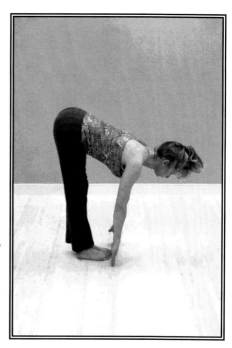

Exhale and step or hop back to **Full Plank (Isa Dandasana)**.

Alignment:

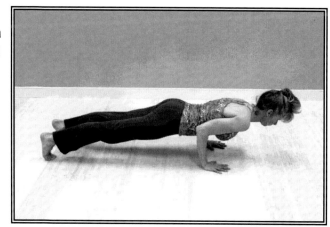

- Shoulders over hands. Draw shoulder blades together and soften through the heart.
- Thigh muscles and abdominals lift and engage.
- Balls of the feet and toes rooted to the earth.
- Optional Modification: Drop the knees to the floor.

Continue to exhale through **Chaturanga Dandasana**, moving from high to low push-up position.

Alignment:

- Arms form 90 degree angles.
- Elbows tucked into the sides grazing the ribcage.
- Abdominal muscles engage and lift.
- Thighs firm and strong.
- Gaze set about 2 feet in front of the fingers.
- Optional Modification: slowly lower the torso to the floor.

Inhale rolling over the toes (**Yogi Toe Roll**) to **Upward Facing Dog** (**Urdhva Mukha Svanasana**).

Alignment:

- Lift and open through the heart.

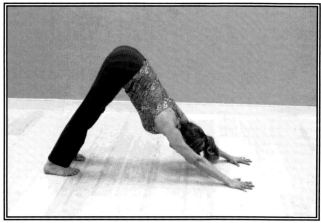

- Press through the hands and tops of the feet.

- Shoulder blades draw together and down the back.

- Gaze forward or upward.

- Optional Modification: release the thighs to the floor, bend the elbows and press lightly through the hands extending through the spine.

Exhale to **Downward Facing Dog (Adho Mukha Svanasana)**.

Alignment:

- Fingers spread wide -ground down through the triads of the hands.

- Draw the shoulder blades down the back and lift through the sitting bones.

- Engage and lift quadriceps.

- Hold for 3 – 5 breaths

- Optional Modification: bend the knees with heels off the floor.

On the final exhalation, empty the lungs and walk, hop or float forward bringing the feet up to meet the hands.

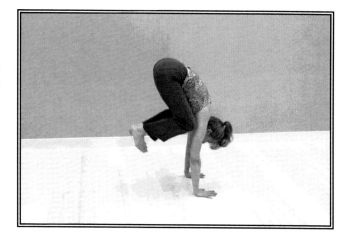

Alignment:

- Hips lift up and then move forward.

- Shoulders aligned over hands.

- Lift up through the belly.

- Gaze 6 – 8 inches in front of the finger tips.

- Optional Modification: Slowly walk the feet up to meet the hands bending and softening through the knees.

Inhale to an **Extended Forward Bend (Urdhva Mukha Uttanasana)**.

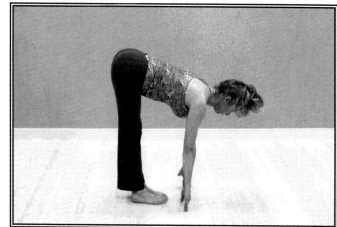

Alignment:

- Maintain a flat back, creating length from the base of the spine to the top of the head.

- Lift and engage the quadriceps.

- Firm and hold the abdominal muscles taut.

- Optional Modification: Bend the knees and rest the hands or fingertips on the shins or thighs.

Exhale to **Forward Bend** (**Uttanasana**).

Alignment:

- Sitting bones reach upward. Hips aligned over heels.

- Torso draped against thighs.

- Soften through the knees, or if flexibility allows, straighten the legs and lift through the knee caps dynamically supporting the thigh muscles.

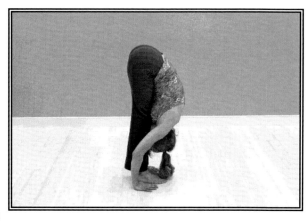

Inhale and press through the feet, engaging the quadriceps and coming through a flat back, **Extended Forward Bend**. Continue inhaling to **Standing Backbend.**

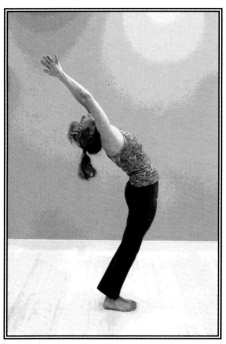

Alignment:

- Fix your feet firmly and tighten through the quadriceps.

- Reach up and back to create length through the entire spinal column.

- Encourage your head to lift up and gently release back.

- Open through the heart and breathe.

- Optional Modification: return to standing **Mountain Pose** with arms reaching overhead.

Exhale to **Mountain Pose**

Alignment:

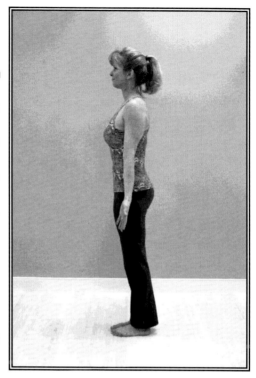

- Connect the feet with the earth - implant the mound under the big and pinky toes and both sides of the heel to the ground.

- Lift through the inner arches of the feet and bring the energy upward into the calf muscles, knees, and thighs.

- The base of the spine (perineum) square to the ground, scooping the pelvic bowl ever so slightly.

- Lift through the heart and release the shoulder blades back and downward.

- Allow the head to rest evenly over the shoulders and set your gaze forward.

Sun Salutation Series B (Surynamaskar B)

Begin in **Tadasana**.

Inhale and extend both arms overhead lowering the buttocks and lifting the torso to **Chair** (**Utkatasana**).

Exhale and fold forward, hinging at the hips and coming through flat back to **Forward Bend** (**Uttanasana**).

Inhale to **Extended Forward Bend** (**Urdhva Mukha Uttanasana**)—maintain a flat back from the base of the spine to the crown of the head.

Exhale step or hop back to **Full Plank** (**Isa Dandasana**). Continue to exhale moving from high push-up to low push-up position (**Chaturanga Dandasana**).

Inhale rolling over the toes to **Upward Facing Dog** (**Urdhva Mukha Svanasana**).

Exhale to **Downward Facing Dog** (**Adho Mukha Svanasana**).

Inhale lifting the right leg behind the body, exhale stepping the right foot forward between the hands. Back heel rotates down to a 45% – 60% angle.

Inhale as you lift the upper body vertical, moving into **Warrior 1** (**Virabhadrasana I**).

Exhale releasing the hands to the floor surrounding the front foot and step the right foot back to **Full Plank** (**Isa Dandasana**). Continue to exhale through **Chaturanga Dandasana**.

Inhale to **Upward Facing Dog** (**Urdhva Mukha Svanasana**).

Exhale to **Downward Facing Dog** (**Adho Mukha Svanasana**).

Repeat on the left side.

Stay in **Downward Facing Dog** for 3 to 5 breaths or longer if needed. On the final exhalation, empty the lungs, and walk or jump forward.

Inhale to **Extended Forward Bend** (**Urdhva Mukha Uttanasana**).

Exhale to **Forward Bend** (**Uttanasana**).

Inhale to **Chair** (**Utkatasana**).

Exhale and return to **Mountain Pose** (**Tadasana**).

Repeat vinyasa 2-4 times.

Sun Salutation Series B (Surynamaskar B)

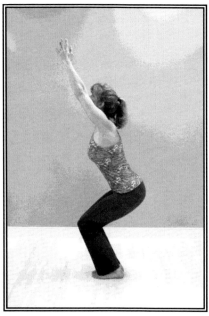

Inhale and extend both arms overhead to **Chair/Thunderbolt (Utkatasana)**.

Alignment:

- Thighs, knees, ankles and feet energetically pressed together.
- Sitting bones reaching for the back wall.
- Lift through the heart and extend the arms, palms facing one another with pinky fingers spinning toward the back wall.
- Soften through the shoulders and release the scapula down the spine.
- Maintain active bandhas.

Exhale fold forward, hinging at the hips to **Extended Forward Bend (Urdhva Mukha Uttanasana)**.

Alignment:

- Reach through the crown of the head, creating length through the entire spinal column.
- Abdominals draw inward toward the spine stabilizing a flat back.
- Fix your feet firmly. Quadriceps lifted and engaged.
- Hands move through heart center or arms extend out to the sides to relieve pressure on the lower back.
- Optional Modification: bend the knees.

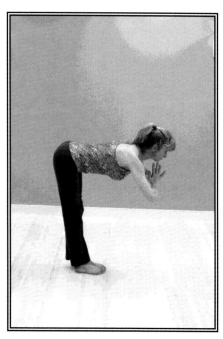

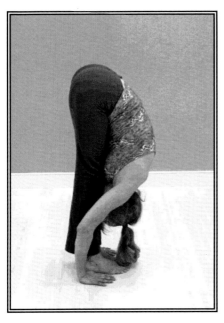

Continue exhaling and empty the lungs to **Forward Bend** (**Uttanasana**).

Alignment:

- Hips aligned over heels.
- Torso draped against thighs.
- Soften through the knees or if flexibility allows, straighten the legs and lift through the knee caps dynamically to engage the thigh muscles.
- Finger tips in line with the toes.
- Optional Modification: bend the knees and rest the hands on the shins or ankles.

Inhale to **Extended Forward Bend** (**Urdhva Mukha Uttanasana**), with a flat back from the base of the spine to the crown of the head.

Alignment:

- Hips aligned over heels.
- Shoulder blades releasing back toward the midline of the body.
- Draw the belly inward.
- Engage and lift thigh muscles.
- Optional Modification: bend the knees and place the hands or fingertips on the thighs or shins.

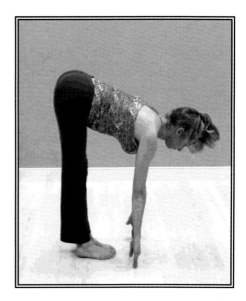

Exhale and step or hop back to **Full Plank (Isa Dandasana)**.

Alignment:

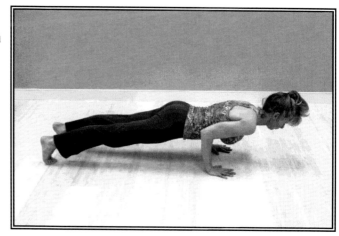

- Shoulders stacked over hands. Shoulder blades draw together and soften through the heart.
- Lift and engage thigh muscles and abdominals.
- Balls of the feet and toes rooted to the earth.
- Optional Modification: Drop the knees to the floor.

Continue to exhale through **Chaturanga Dandasana**, moving from high to low push-up position.

Alignment:

- Arms form 90 degree angles.
- Elbows tucked into the sides grazing the ribcage.
- Engage and lift abdominal muscles.
- Thighs firm and strong.
- Gaze set about 2 feet in front of the fingers.
- Optional Modification: slowly lower the torso to the floor.

Inhale rolling over the toes to **Upward Facing Dog (Urdhva Mukha Svanasana)**.

Alignment:

- Lift and open through the heart.
- Press through the hands and tops of the feet.

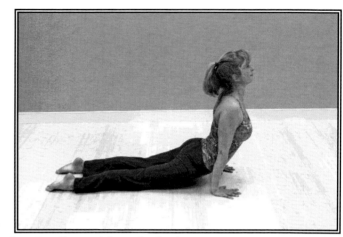

- Shoulder blades draw together and down the back.
- Gaze forward or upward.
- Optional Modification: release the thighs to the floor, bend the elbows and press lightly through the hands extending through the spine.

Exhale to **Downward Facing Dog (Adho Mukha Svanasana)**.

Alignment:

- Fingers spread wide grounding down through the triads of the hands.
- Draw the shoulder blades down the back

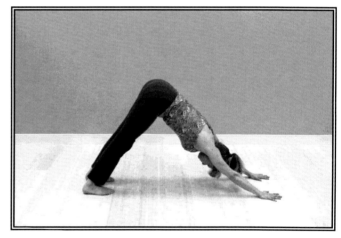

and lift through the sitting bones.
- Engage and lift quadriceps.
- Optional Modification: bend the knees with heels off the floor.

Inhale lifting the right leg behind the body.

Alignment:

- Separate hands shoulder distance width.

- Right leg straight and strong with hips square to the earth.

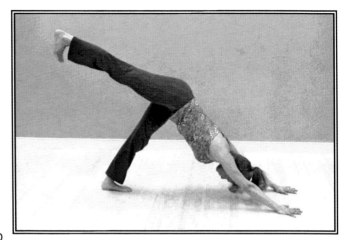

- Active thigh muscles.

- Gaze toward your left big toe.

Exhale and step the right foot forward between the hands. Back heel rotates down to a 45% – 60% angle.

Alignment:

- Hands surround the right foot with fingers aligned near the ankle.

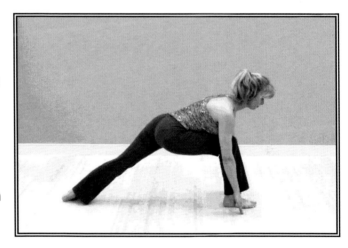

- Drop through the hips and lift through the heart extending the torso over the front leg.

- Back leg firm, planting the outer edge of the left foot to the ground.

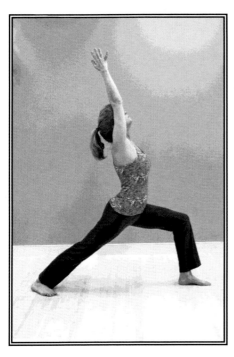

Inhale as you lift the upper body vertical and float into **Warrior 1 (Virabhadrasana I)**

Alignment:

- Head centered over shoulders, shoulders over hips.
- Scoop the pelvic floor forward slightly.
- Engage and straighten through the back leg.
- Release down through the shoulder blades and draw the belly toward the spine.
- Set your gaze forward or allow you eyes to rest at your fingertips.

Exhale and begin releasing the hands toward the floor.

Alignment:

- Extend through the spine and drape the torso over the right leg.
- Maintain abdominal engagement.

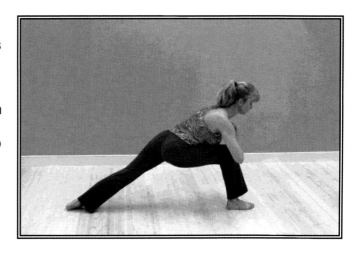

As you exhale surround the front foot and step the right foot back to **Full Plank (Isa Dandasana)**.

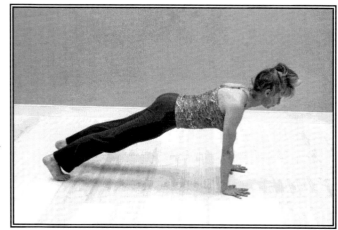

Alignment:

- Shoulder over hands.

- Engage and lift thigh muscles and abdominals.

- Shoulder blades draw together and soften through the heart.

- Balls of the feet and toes rooted to the earth.

- Optional Modification: drop the knees to the floor.

Continue to exhale through **Chaturanga Dandasana**, moving from high to low push-up position.

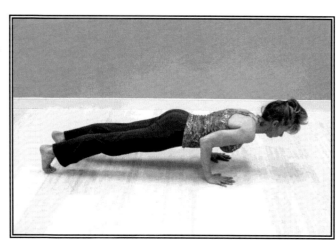

Alignment:

- Arms form 90 degree angles. Elbows tucked into the sides grazing the ribcage

- Engage and lift abdominal muscles.

- Thighs firm and strong.

- Gaze set about 2 feet in front of the fingers.

- Optional Modification: slowly lower the body to the floor.

Begin inhaling and move through a **Yogi Toe Roll.**

Alignment:

- Push through the balls and toes of the feet shifting the body weight forward.

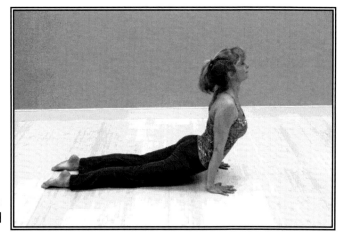

- Maintain firmness through the thighs and abdominals.

- Optional Modification: begin to press into the hands lifting the upper body off the floor.

Complete the inhalation to **Upward Facing Dog (Urdhva Mukha Svanasana).**

Alignment:

- Lift and open through the heart.

- Press through the hands and tops of the feet. Thighs and knees are lifted off the floor.

- Shoulder blades draw together and down the back.

- Gaze forward or upward.

- Optional Modification: keep the hips and thighs resting on the floor and lift the torso. Press lightly into the hands and extend through spine.

Exhale to **Downward Facing Dog** (**Adho Mukha Svanasana**).

Alignment:

- Hands and feet mirror hip and shoulder distance width.

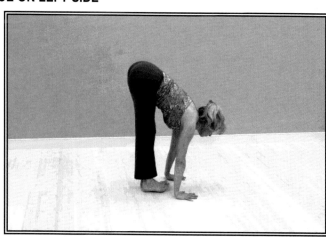

- Draw the shoulder blades down the back and lift through the sitting bones.
- Lift and engage thigh and abdominal muscles.
- Set gaze between your feet.
- Optional Modification: bend the knees with heels off the floor.

REPEAT SEQUENCE ON LEFT SIDE

Stay in **Downward Facing Dog** for 3 to 5 breaths or longer if needed. On the final exhalation, empty the lungs and walk, hop or float forward bringing the feet up to meet the hands.

Alignment:

- Lift hips up and then move forward.
- Shoulders aligned over hands.
- Lift up through the belly
- Gaze 6 – 8 inches in front of your finger tips.
- Optional Modification: Slowly walk the feet forward toward the hands.

Inhale to an extended forward bend (**Urdhva Mukha Uttanasana**).

Alignment:

- Extend through the crown of the head.
- Create length from the base of the spine to the top of the head.

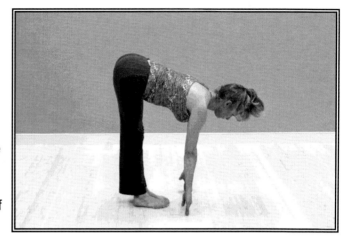

- Engage and lift quadriceps.
- Optional Modification: bend the knees and rest hands on shins

Exhale to **Forward Bend (Uttanasana)**.

Alignment:

- Sitting bones reach upward. Hips aligned over heels.
- Torso draped against thighs.
- Soften through the knees. Or straighten the

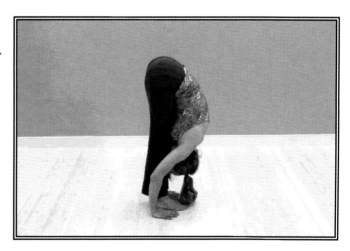

legs and lift through the knee caps dynamically engaging the thigh muscles.

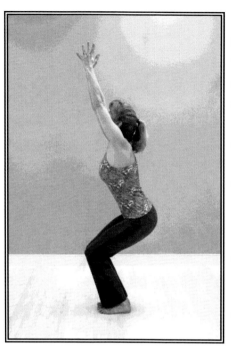

Inhale and extend both arms overhead to **Chair / Thunderbolt (Utkatasana)**.

Alignment:

- Thighs, knees, ankles and feet energetically pressed together.

- Sitting bones reaching for the back wall.

- Lift through the heart and extend arms, palms facing one another with pinky fingers spinning backwards.

- Soften through the shoulders and release the scapula down the spine.

- Engage through the bandhas.

Exhale to **Mountain Pose.**

Alignment:

- Connect the feet with the earth.

- Lift through the inner arches of the feet and bring the energy upward into the calf muscles, knees, and thighs.

- The base of the spine (perineum) square to the ground, scooping the pelvic bowl ever so slightly.

- Lift through the heart and release the shoulder blades back and downward.

- Allow the head to rest evenly over the shoulders and set your gaze forward.

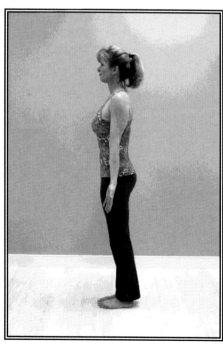

Primary Standing Flow

The **Primary Standing Flow** focuses on developing strength and stamina in both muscles and character. Additional heat is generated by holding and deepening the poses while opening the tension storage areas within the body. We started to tap into the power of breath during the Assessment Series. We stimulated the respiratory system and strengthened cardiovascular ability through the Warm-Up Series. And, now the body is completely warm. We are ready to take the muscles and mind to the next level.

These poses can be quite challenging at times. Power Flow Yoga is designed that way. It is through the effort and level of difficulty that we face our fears, insecurities and preconceived notions. A secure and challenging pose is part of the process. However, there should never be pain. In yoga, pain is pain, not gain. Encourage your physical being to go to its edge but not beyond. The edge is where growth resides. Think about playing the piano. You wouldn't want to play the same song every day. You would want to practice a song until you've mastered it and discovered the flow and beauty of the notes. Once you've done that, you would want to learn a new song and enjoy the process, exploration and resonance of the new experience.

There are numerous asanas that can be used in the standing series, and the type and flow of poses can vary greatly. For our purposes, we will focus on a sequence that provides a well-rounded practice with poses and counter poses. It's basic in its premise and potent in its full expression.

From a physical perspective, Primary Standing Flow builds strong and effective muscles through isometric postures. Physiologically, it will trim fat and tone muscles. As the gaze or drishti comes to rest, the mind will settle and the body will begin to open. Mentally, participants may be challenged and resist the stillness of holding the asanas. This challenge is an integral and necessary experience in yoga. It is the basis from which the individual practice will grow. Tune into the breath observe your thoughts. Let the mind wrestle a bit and focus on the Ujjayi pranayama to find the calm within the storm.

One-Yoga practice is a physical, mental and spiritual process. As we challenge the body and mind, the ego is forced to surrender and step aside. Once the ego is submissive, the emotions and spirit of each practice will surface.

Transition: Do half of **Sun Salutation B** until you come to **Warrior 1** pose.

Pose 5: Warrior 1 (Virabhadrasana I)

Right leg is bent at approximately a 90-degree angle. Back leg is engaged and straight with outer edges of the foot and pinky toe pressing down. Scoop the tailbone forward slightly. Reach up with the arms and relax down through the shoulder blades. Hands are active. Continue to straighten through the elbows while moving the shoulders away from the ears. The upper body should be light and energized--centered between the legs. The lower body is solid, stable and strong. Drishti: the finger tips or a spot directly in front of the eyes.

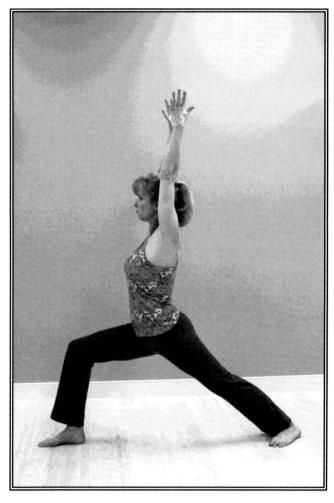

HOLD FOR 5 BREATHS

Transition: Inhale fully and as you exhale open up the arms and hips to **Warrior 2** pose.

Pose 6: Warrior 2 (Virabhadrasana II)

Right leg remains bent at a 90-degree angle. Keep the knee centered over the ankle, engaging through the inner thigh and quadriceps. Hips are now open to the side. Think about rotating the right inner thigh up and to the right, while simultaneously rotating the left inner thigh up and out to the left. Back leg is straight and strong, with outer edges of the foot and pinky toe pressing down. Center the upper body evenly between the legs and find the balance in this dynamic pose. Scoop the tailbone forward slightly engaging through Mulabandha and bringing the pelvic floor to face the earth. Arms extend out over the legs. Relax down through the shoulder blades. Hands are active. Drishti: over the right middle or index finger.

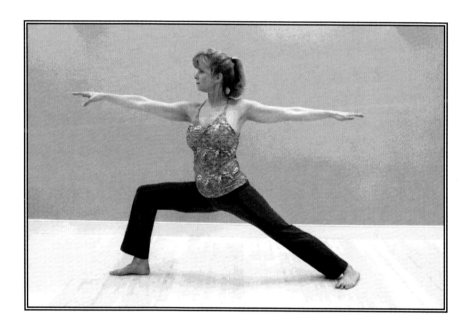

HOLD FOR 5 BREATHS

Transition: While inhaling, flip the palm of the right hand and reach upward. Sink into the front knee and extend the upper body to **Reverse Warrior** pose.

Pose 7: Reverse Warrior (Parivrtta Virabhadrasana)

Right leg remains bent at a 90-degree angle. The thigh muscles may be challenged and shaky as you sink into the legs and tap into the fire, but stay present and foster the new muscle memory. Keep the knee centered over the ankle. Extend up through the right side of the torso creating length and space between hip joint and ribcage. Outstretched arm is active with fingertips reaching up and slightly back. The lower body remains the same. Back hand reaches down the left leg--energized and extending. Do not press on the back knee for support. Drishti: right thumb

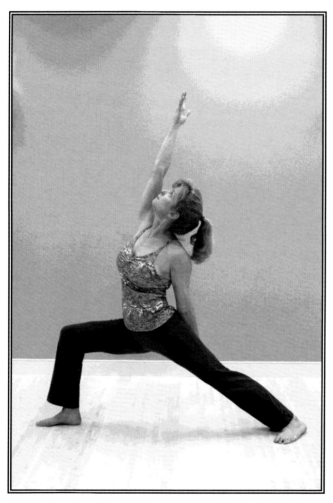

HOLD FOR 5 BREATHS

Transition: While exhaling, place the right forearm on the right thigh, moving into **Extended Side Angle**.

Pose 8: Extended Side Angle (Utthita Parsvakonasana)

Right leg remains bent at a 90-degree angle. Drop through the hips and press through the outer edge of the left foot. The back leg serves as an anchor as you draw the inner thigh (adductor) into the body. Keep the right knee centered over the ankle. Left arm reaches straight up to the ceiling. Left shoulder should be aligned over top of the right. If hip flexibility allows, lower the right hand to clasp the right ankle or place the hand to the inside of the right foot, reach the left hand forward, palm facing the earth. Rotate the heart upward and draw the shoulder blades together and down the back. Extension along the entire left side of the body is a key aspect of this pose. The body, left foot to head should be on a diagonal line. Drishti: left fingertips, left bicep or a spot on the ceiling.

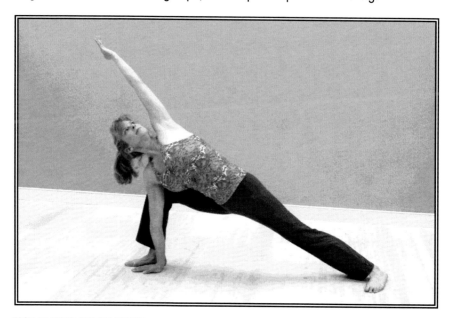

HOLD FOR 5 BREATHS

Transition: On an inhalation, lift the torso and return to **Warrior 2**. Exhale and settle into the pose. Inhale and completely stabilize the pose. Exhale and release both arms to the floor, surrounding the right foot. Step back to **High or Full Plank** position. Inhale in **High Plank (Isa Dandasana)**; exhale moving from High Plank to low push-up position (**Chaturanga Dandasana**); inhale moving through a (**Yogi Toe Roll**) to **Upward Facing Dog**; and exhale to **Downward Facing Dog**. This is also known as half of a vinyasa. Repeat Poses 5, 6, 7, and 8 with transition on the left side. Go through half of a vinyasa and ride the breath to standing **Mountain** pose **(Tadasana).**

Pose 9: Chair/Thunderbolt (Utkatasana)

From **Mountain** pose, with knees, feet, and thighs energetically pressing together, inhale while lowering hips to a seated chair position and bring arms extending overhead at a 45-degree angle. Engage through the abdominal region. Imagine the belly button being pulled slightly to the spine. Relax through the shoulders, allowing them to move away from the ears drawing the base of the scapula together. Drishti: gaze at the fingertips or a spot directly in front of you.

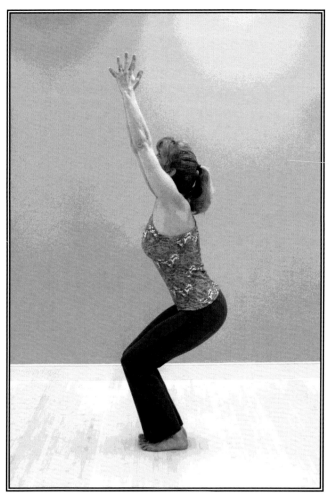

HOLD FOR 5 BREATHS

Transition: Exhale and fold forward, releasing the pose to open the sacral area. Separate the feet about two fists' distance (approximately hip width) and move into **Gorilla** pose.

Pose 10: Gorilla Pose / Hand-to-Big Toe Forward Bend (Padangusthasana)

Feet remain in hip width stance, approximately 6 to 8 inches apart. Soften through the knees so that the torso rests on the thighs. Clasp a yogi toe lock-- index and middle finger slide between the big toe and second toe, and thumb wraps around the inside edge of the big toe. Inhale to an **Extended Forward Bend** position--flat back (**Urdhva Mukha Uttanasana**), lifting the toe lock. While exhaling, fold forward and bring the head between the legs, abdominals engaged and lifted. Strive to straighten the legs as much as the hamstrings will allow, dynamically lifting through the knee caps. Root down through the big toe and the padded mounds under the big and small toes. Keep breathing deeply and try to give into the gravitational pull of the pose. Drishti: gaze at the bellybutton or tip of the nose.

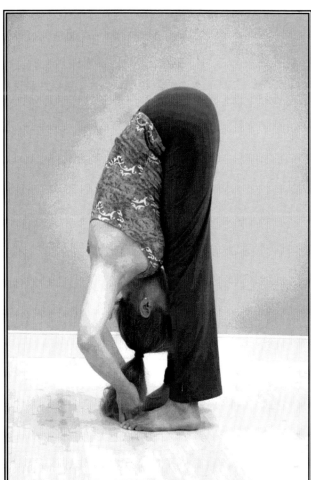

HOLD FOR 5 BREATHS

Transition: Inhale and release the toe lock, extending forward to flat back position. Exhale and toe-heel the feet and legs together folding forward. Inhale, releasing the buttocks and sitting bones downward, extending the arms overhead to **Chair/ Thunderbolt** pose in preparation for the next pose.

Pose 11: Revolved Chair/Prayer Twist (Parivrtta Utkatasana)

Start in **Chair/Thunderbolt** pose, with knees, feet and thighs energetically pressed together. Exhale and bring the hands into prayer position at heart center. With a flat back, rotate the torso to the right. Initiate the action from the lower abdominal area first, following with the ribcage and upper chest. Bring the left triceps muscle to the right thigh and leverage the twist using the arms as well as the abdominals. Work to keep the knees and hips facing forward, actively extending through the spine, elongating from the crown of the head to the base of the sacrum. Drishti: set the gaze up, or flower the arms open and gaze at the fingertips.

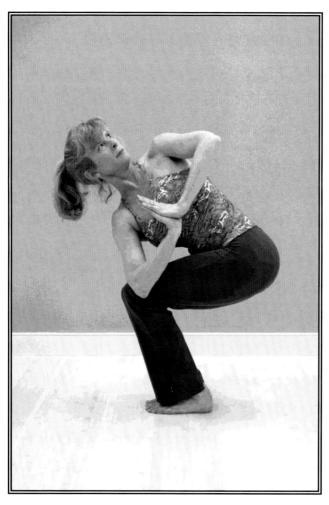

HOLD FOR 5 BREATHS

Transition: Inhale and return the torso forward. Exhale and fold forward, releasing the pose to open the sacral and lower lumbar areas. Separate the feet about two fists' distance apart (approximately hip width) and move into a deeper variation of **Gorilla** pose.

Pose 12: Gorilla Pose / Hand-to-Foot Forward Bend (Padahastasana)

Feet remain in hip width stance, approximately 6 to 8 inches apart. Soften through the knees so the torso rests on the thighs. Slide the hands under the feet palms up, so that the toes are draped on the wrists. Inhale to an extended forward bend position with **Flat Back (Urdhva Uttanasana)**, applying pressure and weight to the hands. While exhaling, fold forward and bring the head between the legs, abdominals engaged and lifted. Strive to straighten the legs as much as the hamstrings will allow – dynamically lifting through the knee caps. Continue to breathe deeply and energize the quadriceps. Drishti: gaze at the bellybutton, base of spine or tip of the nose.

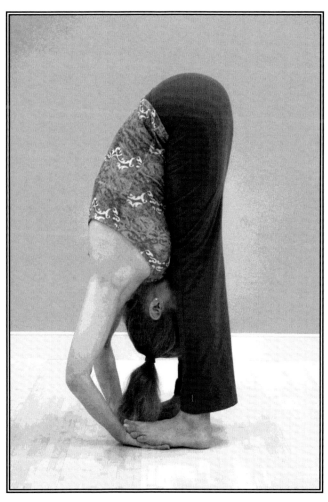

HOLD FOR 5 BREATHS

Transition: Inhale and release the pose, extending forward to flat back position. Exhale and toe-heel the feet and legs together folding forward. Inhale, releasing the buttocks and sitting bones to a seated position, extending the arms overhead to **Chair/ Thunderbolt** pose. Repeat pose 11 on the left side.

Transition: Inhale and return the torso forward. Exhale and fold forward, releasing the pose to open the sacral and lower lumbar areas. Keep the feet together in preparation for our next variation of **Forward Bend** pose.

Pose 13: Hand to Heel Extended Forward Bend Pose (Utthita Hasta Padagohira Uttanasana)

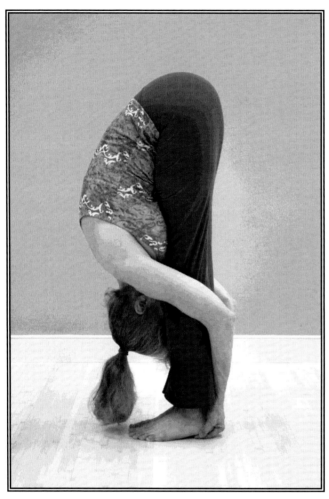

Feet are together with toes and heels touching. Soften through the knees so the torso rests on the thighs. Slide the hands under the heels palms up. In this position, the heels will be stepping on the fingers and palms. Or place the fingertips at the base of the ankles. Bring the forearms behind the calf muscles so that the ulna or back sides of the forearms and elbows are working to come together – wrists touching. Inhale lengthening through the spine as much as possible. Exhale deepening the forward fold. Engage and lift through the thighs. Breathe fully and begin to straighten the legs as much as possible without separating the torso from the thighs. Encourage the base of the spine and sacral area to spread and open. Drishti: Tip of the nose.

HOLD FOR 5-10 BREATHS

Transition: Inhale, releasing the pose. Exhale and interlace the fingers, extending the index fingers encouraging them to reach forward and touch the ground 6 to 8 inches in front of the feet. Inhale releasing the buttocks and sitting bones to a **Chair** position. Continue inhaling – coming through flat back and reach the arms fully overhead. Exhale and return to **Mountain Pose.** Take a moment – breathe and allow your body to absorb the practice so far – refocus your mind and revisit intention.

Secondary Standing Flow

The **Secondary Standing Flow** concentrates on accessing deeper muscles of the hips, legs and torso. Balancing, revolving and hip oriented standing poses are introduced. Appropriate alignment and listening to your body are important to ensure safety and derive the physiological benefits.

Initiating and sustaining poses that access the surrounding and supporting muscles of the hips may meet with resistance. The hips are like an axis. Both upper and lower body mobility is united and somewhat dependent on hip flexibility. Stay with the breath. The Ujjayi pranayama will help you channel your attention to explore the physical, mental and emotional benefits of these poses. When muscles start to tremble or shake, just keep breathing. Allow your eyes to rest on a focal point and tune into the deep rhythmical breath of Ujjayi. This sequencing of poses is structured to prepare the body and mind for depths of spiritual awakening that arises from hip-opening asanas.

In the beginning there is breath (Assessment Series), which invites us into the present moment. Life begins to move and generate energy (Warm-Up Series). Strength, stamina and confidence are cultivated as we grow and learn to use our power (Primary Standing Flow). Now, we are ready to move on and begin to unleash the aptitude locked in the histories of our body. Many passageways lead to self-realization and fulfillment. My experience has shown that our hips serve as stress repositories. The **Secondary Standing Flow** begins to open those stress centers and guides our understanding through the practice of several basic and potent asanas.

Transition: Do half of **Sun Salutation A** until you come to **Downward Facing Dog** pose. Inhale and lift your right leg keeping the hips square to the earth. Exhale using your core strength to step the right foot between the hands. Leave the left heel spun up staying on the ball of the foot.

Pose 14: Crescent Lunge (Anjaneyasana)

Inhale raising the torso vertical – centered between the legs. Right leg is bent at a 90-degree angle. Back leg is engaged and lifted. Work to straighten the back knee as you press the ball of the foot into the earth – heel up and pressing back. Root the strength of this pose between both legs and find balance. Scoop the tailbone forward slightly. Reach up with the arms and relax down through the shoulder blades. Continue to straighten through the elbows while moving the shoulders away from the ears. Hands are active. Palms touching or hands and arms shoulder distance width. Drishti: gaze at the thumbs or forward resting the eyes on a spot.

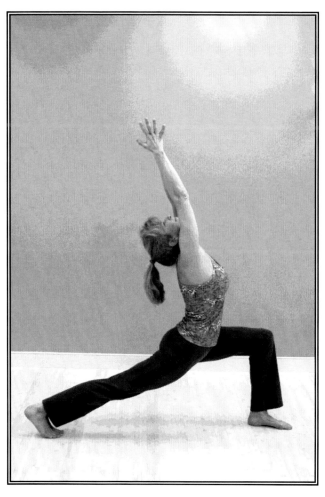

HOLD FOR 5 BREATHS

Transition: On an exhalation bring the hands in heart center in prayer position in preparation for **Revolved Crescent Lunge**.

Pose 15: Revolved Crescent Lunge (Parivrtta Alanasana)

Inhale and lift through the sternum drawing the shoulder blades together down the back. Exhale and rotate the torso to the right. Lengthen through the entire spinal column twisting from the navel. Use left triceps as a lever pressing into the right thigh to extend the spine and rotate the front of the body – heart moving upward. Right leg maintains 90-degree angle. Secure the stability of this pose by engaging the back leg and pressing down through the padded mounds under the big and pinky toes. Palms together at heart center or flower the arms open bringing the left fingertips to the outer edge of the right foot. Drishti: set the gaze up, or focus on the extended fingertips.

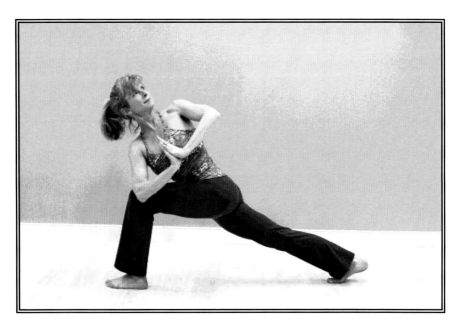

HOLD FOR 5 BREATHS

Transition: On an inhalation return to **Crescent Lunge.**

Pose 16: Intense Side Stretch /
Bowing Warrior Pose (Parsvottanasana)

Exhale and straighten the legs. Step the back foot in about 12 inches. Inhale reaching through the fingertips and lifting through the spine. Exhale hinging at the hips. Drape the upper body over the extended right leg. Internally pull the right thigh back and left thigh forward, creating a scissor effect. Engage the quadriceps and adductor muscles. Hips are square. As flexibility allows, place fingertips or palms on the floor to externally support the upper body. Advanced practioners can interlace fingers – extending index fingers slightly out in front of the right foot, and bringing the forehead to rest on the knee or shin. Drishti: gaze at the big toe or knee, maintaining spinal alignment.

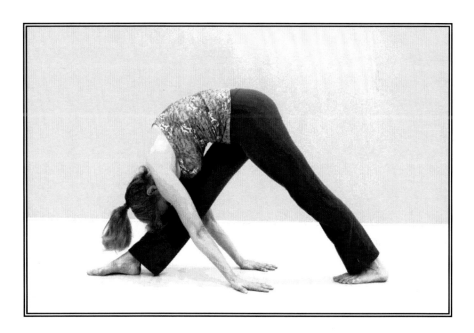

HOLD FOR 5 BREATHS

Transition: Soften the right leg bending the knee and begin to shift weight forward. Place both hands 6 to 8 inches in front of the right foot and come to a standing balance on the right leg.

Pose 17: Half Moon Pose (Ardha Chandrasana)

From a standing balance on the right leg, begin to open the hips, stacking the left hip on top of the right. Align right thumb approximately 6 to 8 inches out in front of the right pinky toe. Come to claw like finger tips and lengthen through the spine. Engage the thigh muscles of both legs and root down through the four corners of the standing foot. Legs are straight and active. Left foot should be flexed with the knee and toes facing the side. Release the left hand to the base of the sacrum and begin to open the torso to the left. Inhale as you reach up with the left arm stacking the shoulders. Expose the heart, and allow your gaze to rise up. Drishti: Eyes rest forward, toward the left thumb or a spot on the ceiling.

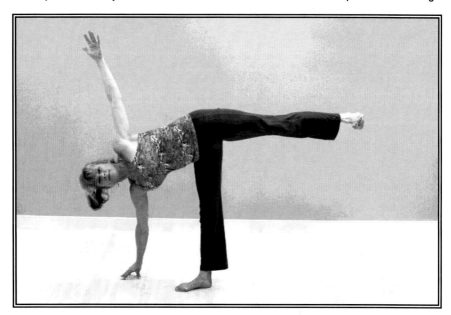

HOLD FOR 5 BREATHS

Transition: Exhale, releasing the pose by squaring the hips and bringing the left foot down to meet the right in a forward bend position. Inhale and bend into the knees lowering the buttocks and move to **Chair / Thunderbolt** pose. Exhale to **Mountain** pose. Go through half of a vinyasa. Repeat Poses 14, 15, 16, and 17 with transition on the left side. Go through half of a vinyasa and ride the breath to standing **Mountain** pose (**Tadasana**).

Balancing Asanas

Balancing Asanas promote mindfulness and awareness. They enable conscious perception of our being. Both symmetrical and asymmetrical balancing poses reveal strength, weakness, balance, and imbalance in our physical, mental and emotional states. Balancing poses foster concentration and mental clarity. They are demanding and invigorating. Give yourself permission to be non-judgmental. Don't think. Just tap into the rhythm of your breath and investigate these poses. Maintaining the flow of pranayama provides a foundation for exploring and absorbing the power behind these postures.

Throughout our life's journey we encounter obstacles. We may have been injured or experienced emotional trauma. We may have been functioning day to day on the treadmill of western society. We may have relationship issues or suffer from disabilities. This can all contribute to the imbalance that is inherent in our culture. Balancing poses will enlighten our awareness of static and dynamic equilibrium while fostering composure and peace.

Through the process of life, energy, strength, and opening, we are guided to understand the importance of balance. In the **Balancing Asanas,** we will explore the opportunity of overcoming blockages that prevent harmony. There are many wonderful balancing postures. This practice will focus on three.

Pose 18: Crow Pose (Bakasana)

From **Mountain** pose, standing at the top of the mat, separate the feet to the edges of the mat. Inhale reaching arms overhead. Exhale lowering the hips to the floor between the legs, coming into a **yogi squat**. Place the hands on the floor, shoulder distance apart about 12 inches in front of feet. (Arms are forming shelves for the knees to rest on) Inhale as the hips are lifted into the air. Exhale and position the knees on the triceps or even higher into the armpits and shift the weight into the hands. Bring the big toes to touch behind the buttocks. Pull the bellybutton in toward the spine as the back is rounded. Drishti: gaze at the floor or if stable begin to set the eyes forward.

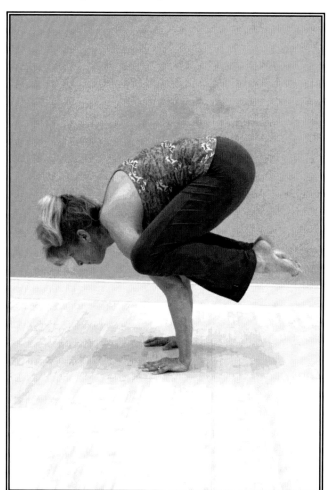

HOLD FOR 5 BREATHS

Transition: Exhale, releasing the pose. Return to a yogi squat position and step back or shoot the legs out behind, coming into **Full Plank**. Proceed through half of a vinyasa and ride the breath to standing **Mountain** pose, with hands at heart center prayer position.

Pose 19: Eagle Pose (Garudasana)

From **Mountain** pose, inhale and bring arms overhead. Exhale, opening arms to the sides and begin double wrapping the arms, right under the left and palms touching. Lift the elbows shoulder level, press the hands forward and release the shoulder blades down the back. Bend both knees and cross right leg over the left, or if flexibility permits, double wrap legs. Sit down low into the pose, keeping the head centered over shoulders, shoulders stacked over hips and hips centered over feet. Maintain core awareness—keep the abdominals slightly taut. Slow the breath. Drishti: fix the gaze forward or at the tip of the nose.

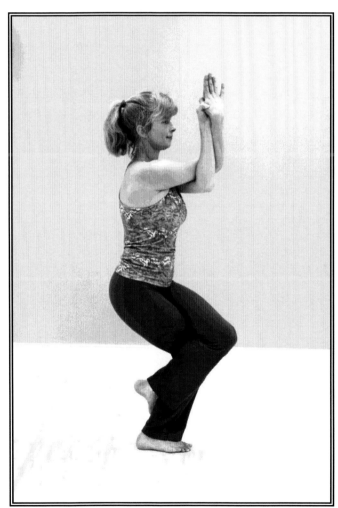

HOLD FOR 5 BREATHS

Transition: Inhale and release the pose, arms moving downward and then reaching up, as though coming out of water. Exhale and repeat **Eagle** pose on the left side. Left arm wraps under right and left leg over right.

HOLD FOR 5 BREATHS

Repeat Eagle and Transition one more time each side. Transition: Lower the right hand down and keep the left arm extended overhead in preparation for **Dancer's** pose.

Pose 20: Dancer's Pose (Natarajasana)

Bend the right knee with the heel of the right foot reaching for the right buttock. With the right hand, reach back and grab the inner arch of the right foot. Knees should be as close together as possible for the beginning of this pose. Tilt the pelvic bowl forward with the spine upright and aligned. You may feel a nice quadriceps stretch. Extend and reach forward with the left arm. Slowly start to kick the right foot into the right hand. Use the strength of the kick to lift the leg into the air away from the buttocks. (This is the beginning of the back-bending series, so there will be a slight stretch in the lower back). Allow the kicking action of the foot to open the shoulder and rotator cuff. Keep breathing slow and rhythmically—keep

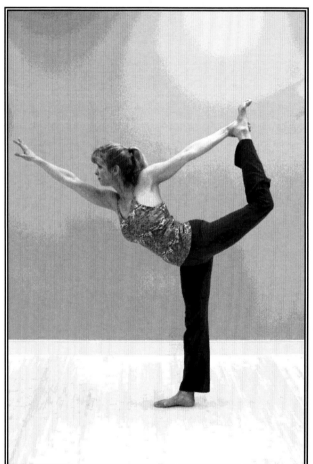

kicking and lift and open the heart.
Drishti: Finger tips, straight ahead or a spot on the floor.

HOLD FOR 5 BREATHS

Transition: Windmill the arms and repeat the sequence on the left side.
Repeat one more time each side.

Transition: Go through a full **Sun Salutation A**, ending in **Downward Facing Dog**. Inhale to **High Plank** and lower slowly to the floor in a prone position.

Back-Bending Series

Back-bending postures serve the body in many ways. Effective and safe back-bending postures are used to increase flexibility, strength and blood supply to the trunk of the body. They are vital to the overall health and well-being of an individual because they strengthen the muscles surrounding the spinal column. A strong back reinforces postural alignment. Increased blood flow to the spinal area benefits the nervous system through nerve stimulation. Back bends stretch the abdominal area and assist with digestion as they tone abdominal muscles and digestive organs. Back bends are usually associated with the opening and exposure of the solar plexus area. Increasing blood supply and activity to the solar plexus energy center can exert a chemical influence on the stomach, liver and spleen.

There is often an emotional reluctance that surfaces in back-bending postures. That's because these poses completely expose the internal organs—most importantly, the heart. Many experience a sense of vulnerability both physically and emotionally. Permitting the heart to open and relinquishing control over all the details of our lives is good – scary, but good. As thoughts arise, turn the consciousness to breath. Listen and feel the breath as it enters and exits the body.

As one who has experienced lower back issues, be mindful. Back off if there is pain. When the feeling is slight discomfort, it may present an opportunity to breathe through the pose and begin the process of healing. The body is beginning to open up and the struggle may be more than physical – it may be internal. As humans, we go to great lengths to avoid discomfort. It is innate for us to seek pleasure and avoid dismay. As we work through our fears and anguish associated with back bending poses the guarding of the heart melts away.

We have progressed through our yoga practice much like we do through our lives. And through this progression, we have learned to protect our heart. We now have rediscovered the importance of balance and are led to a place that shows us the significance of being open and receptive. In order to move to the next step we will strengthen our spines – the supporting structure of our being and expose our heart the muscle responsible for life – courage, compassion and love.

Pose 21: Cobra Pose (Bhujangasana)

This pose can be performed in several different ways depending on back strength and flexibility. Here is one variation.

Place hands flat on the floor, palms down, alongside the lower portion of the ribcage. Legs and feet are close together with inner thighs spiraling in and upward. Press down through the tops of the feet and lift the knees off the floor. Pull the elbows back toward the midline of the spine and release the shoulder blades down the back moving toward the buttocks. Inhale, lifting the heart and chest off the floor (hands can hover just above the floor). Keep extending through the legs, upper back and neck. Drishti: set eyes approximately two feet out in front on the floor – as though gazing at the horizon.

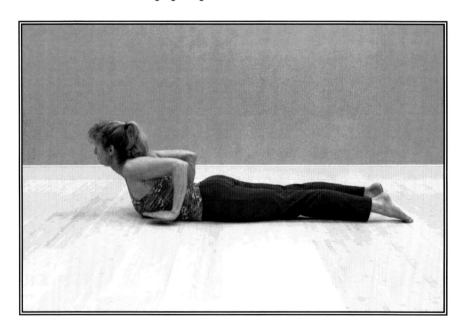

HOLD FOR 5 BREATHS

Transition: Exhale and release the pose, coming into rest. Bring big toes together, splay the heels apart, arms by the sides, and turn the head over the right shoulder pressing the left ear into the floor. Take rest for two complete breaths.

Pose 22: Locust Pose (Salabhasana)

This pose can also be performed in several different ways. Here is one variation.

Bring chin or forehead straight forward, touching the mat. Move hands, palms down, flat on the floor underneath the pelvis. Arms are straight, elbows tucked in. The pinky fingers of the hands, wrists and forearms are working to touch each other. Bring the feet together, toes and heels touching. Maintain straight legs with the inner thighs spiraling inward and upward. Tuck the chin slightly, extending the spine while pressing through the hands and arms. Inhale and exhale while lifting the legs as one unit. Drishti: tip of the nose or floor.

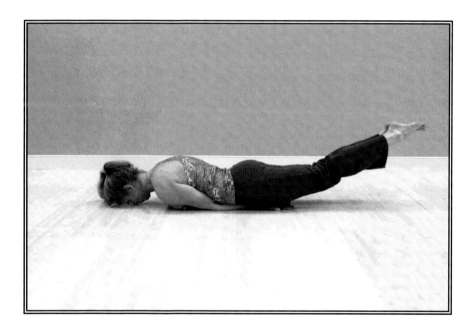

HOLD FOR 5 BREATHS

Transition: Exhale and release the pose coming into rest. Bring big toes together, splay the heels apart, release the arms by the sides, palms up, and turn the head over the left shoulder, pressing the right ear into the floor. Take rest for two complete breaths.

Pose 23: Bow Pose (Dhanurasana)

Bring chin straight forward touching the mat. Lie on the stomach and bend the knees. Reach back and grab the feet or ankles, with hands on the outside of the ankle bones. Bring the knees and feet together as close as possible. Strive for no further then hip width. Inhale and lift the heart and chest off the floor. While exhaling, kick through the legs, lifting the thighs off the floor. Extend and relax through the neck. Drishti: gaze at a spot on the floor 2 – 3 feet in front of the head or straight ahead – as though gazing at the horizon.

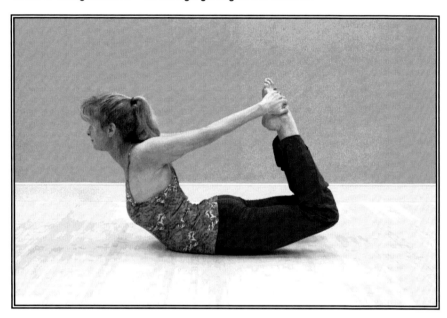

HOLD FOR 5 BREATHS

Transition: Exhale and release the pose coming into rest. Bring big toes together, splay the heels apart, arms by the sides, and turn the head over the right shoulder pressing the left ear into the floor. Take rest for two complete breaths. Repeat the pose once more and alternate the resting gaze. To move into the next pose, **Camel**, begin with chin facing forward touching the mat. Bring hands under shoulders, palms pressing into the earth. Lift the sitting bones and press into the hands. Come to tabletop position—knees positioned under hips and hands under shoulders. Inhale and stand on the knees.

Pose 24: Camel Pose (Ustrasana)

Start with the knees separated, about hip distance apart. Root down through the tops of the feet and press the shins into the floor. Press the hips forward until thighs are perpendicular to the floor and scoop the pelvic floor down and forward. Bring the hands to the base of the spine, fingertips facing upward. Pull the elbows in toward the midline of the back and release the shoulder blades down. Extend through the neck and lift through the sternum, exposing the heart center upward. If flexibility and comfort allow, exhale as the head is released back and place the hands on the heels. Inhale and exhale and release to this heart-pumping back-bend pose. Drishti: upward or at a spot on the floor.

HOLD FOR 5 BREATHS

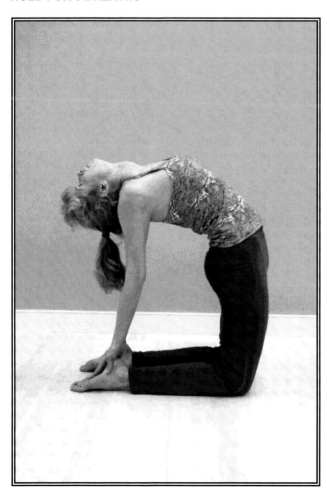

Transition: Inhale and rise up coming out of the pose allowing the head to be the last thing to return to neutral position. Exhale and move to **Tabletop** pose. Inhale curl toes under. Exhale and lift sitting bones high moving into **Downward Facing Dog** pose. Hold transitional pose for 3 breaths and return to knees for second set of **Camel** pose.

Repeat transition. From **Downward Facing Dog**, move through half a vinyasa and sit on the floor setting up for our next pose – **Bridge**.

Pose 25: Bridge Pose (Setubandhasana)

Lie on the back. Bend the knees with feet flat on the floor, close to buttocks. Feet hip width apart and parallel. Stack the knees directly over the ankles. Press evenly through the four corners of the feet encouraging the mound under the big toe to root solidly down. Inhale while lifting the hips. Exhale and gently arch the back while inching the shoulders together underneath the body. Interlace the hands under the body or place them at the sides or on the ankles. Inhale, exhale and release the buttocks as much as possible – lifting the hips and heart up. Move the chin away from the collarbone creating space and permitting the natural curvature of the cervical spine. Drishti: heart center or tip of the nose.

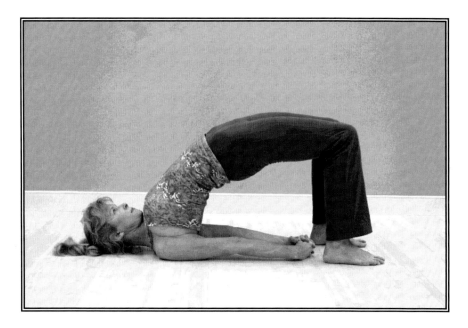

HOLD FOR 5 BREATHS

Transition: Exhale and release the spine to the floor one vertebra at a time, starting with the neck and moving down to the sacrum. Engage the core muscles pressing the lower lumbar into the earth. Hold for two breaths.

Pose 26: One Leg Shoulder Bridge Pose (Ekapada Setubhugasana)

Inhale and return to **Bridge** pose. Use the hands for support under the lower lumbar area if needed. Or, interlace hands under the body or place them on the floor, palms down. Press through the arms and left foot, grounding the connection to the earth. Exhale and release the right leg straight up. Hold the pose inhaling and exhaling to develop strength, stamina and character. Be conscious of neck alignment and keep space between the base of the neck and the floor, lengthening through the crown of the head. Drishti: belly button or tip of the nose.

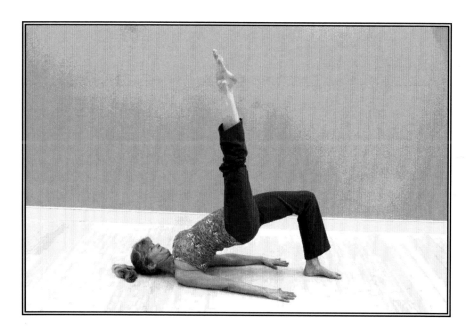

HOLD FOR 5 BREATHS

Transition: Exhale and release the spine to the floor one vertebra at a time, starting with the neck and moving down to the sacrum. Engage the core muscles pressing the lower lumbar into the earth. Hold for two breaths. Repeat the pose and transition on opposite leg.

Pose 27: Wheel Pose (Urdhva Dhanurasana)

Start with feet hip width apart. Root down evenly through the feet. Stack the knees over the heels. Flip the hands with palms on the floor, fingertips facing the feet and hands under the shoulders. Bring the elbows toward each other at shoulder width distance. Drop the shoulder blades down the back before lifting. When inhaling, begin to lift and come to the crown of the head. Tuck in the elbows and shoulders before full extension. Exhale and lift up to full wheel or backbend pose. Focus on the four points touching the earth while lifting the hips and releasing the neck. Press through the hands and extend the elbows. Connect through the padded mounds under the big and little toes and evenly through the heels. Relax and breathe. Drishti: fingertips or a spot on the floor between the hands.

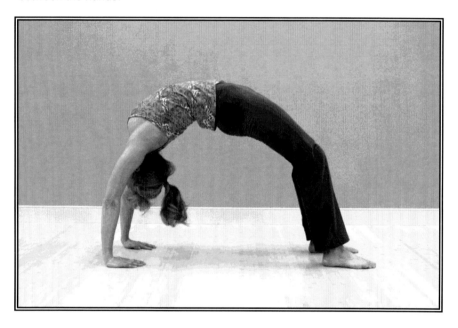

HOLD FOR 5 BREATHS

Transition: Exhale and begin to come out of the pose tucking chin to chest. Release head, neck, shoulders and spine one vertebra at a time. Engage the core muscles pressing the lower lumbar into the earth. Hold for two breaths. Repeat **Wheel** pose and transition. Inhale as you bend the knees and lift both legs in the air.

Core Work

During this portion of practice we will focus on the core area of our body involving the torso, abdominals, and hip flexor regions. An integral part of maintaining overall health involves strengthening our core muscles.

Exercises involving the abdominal area of the body generate heat and stimulate respiratory activity. The abs and hip flexors also serve as opposing muscle groups to the back. When you work opposing muscle groups, it promotes balance of tissue strength and development, and brings neutrality back to the nervous system and spine.

Equilibrium is brought to the physical muscular skeletal system by working both the front and the back of the body. Throughout the practice, core muscles are called into use. However, it is beneficial to implement core-focused poses as counter poses to back bending work. A word of caution: it is my experience that moving from one extreme to another is difficult, even for advanced practiioners. After completing the back bending work it is best to transition to core exercises using a stabilizing posture such as the lumbar press, downward facing dog or plank position. A vinyasa (sun salutation A) is always a nice option as well.

We direct attention to the rectus abdominis, internal and external oblique muscles, and hip flexor areas of the body. The emphasis on **core work** stimulates heat, activity and blood flow in preparation for our hip-opening and closing sequences. There are numerous exercises and poses that can be utilized in this portion of the practice. For our purposes, we will focus on three basic and effective asanas.

Pose 28: Drawbridge (Adhara Bandhasana)

Feet are flexed, big toes touching and positioned directly over the hips forming a 90 degree angle with the upper body. Inhale and press the lower lumbar into the ground, dynamically engaging through the abdominals and quadriceps. While exhaling, lift the head, neck and shoulders a few inches off the floor while lowering the legs on an 8 count. Stop when heels hover about 12 inches off the floor or when the lower lumbar begins to lose its contact with the earth. Palms face each other suspended above the floor, or face down supporting the lower back. Drishti: big toes

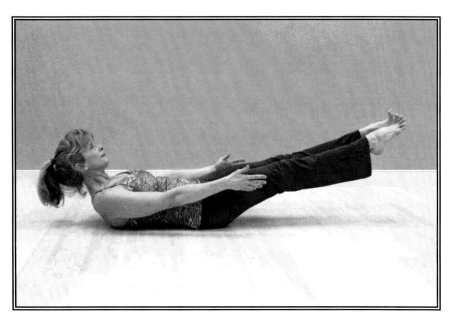

HOLD FOR 3 BREATHS

Transition: Inhale and bend the knees into the chest. Straighten legs upward, returning to 90 degree position. Optional: Inhale with straight legs returning them on an 8 count to 90 degree position. Repeat sequence 2 more times. Complete the **drawbridge** hugging knees to chest. Release knees, placing feet flat on the floor.

Pose 29: Moving Eagle (Acopaca Garudasana)

Inhale and open the arms out to the sides at shoulder height. Exhale and begin to come into a reclined **Eagle** pose. Right arm double wraps under left. Elbows are lifted away from the belly button, palms reaching away from the face. Cross the right leg over the left. If flexibility permits, double wrap legs, hooking the right toes down by the left ankle. Align the spine so that all vertebrae are touching the earth. Maintain the spinal contact throughout the movement. Inhale, as fingertips reach and touch overhead while left heel or toes touch the earth about 12 inches away from buttocks. Exhale and fold the body together. Knees and elbows meet lifting the hips slightly off the floor. Inhale and release fingertips and heel to touch the earth. Drishti: inner eye of the elbow

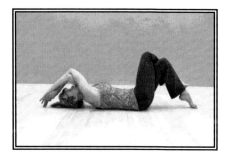 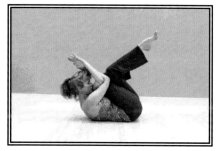

REPEAT 10 TIMES

Transition: Inhale and release the pose - stretch the body out in a five point star. Take rest for two breaths. Exhale and repeat **Moving Eagle** pose on the left side. Left arm wraps under right and left leg over right.

REPEAT 10 TIMES

Transition: Inhale and release the pose - stretch the body out in a five point star. Take rest for two breaths. Exhale hugging knees into the chest. Rock and roll forward and backward until coming to a seated position. Rest on the sitting bones.

Pose 30: Boat Pose (Navasana)

Start seated while lifting through the heart. Back is straight, abdominals are engaged. Imagine pulling the belly button toward the spine. Inhale while lifting the legs into a V or boat position. Exhale and balance on the sitting bones. Lift through the heart and draw the shoulder blades together medially. Legs are straight and engaged, toes spread wide. Arms are extended. Palms are facing each other, fingers energized. Modification: Bend the knees and/or support the lower back with hands behind the buttocks. Drishti: big toes

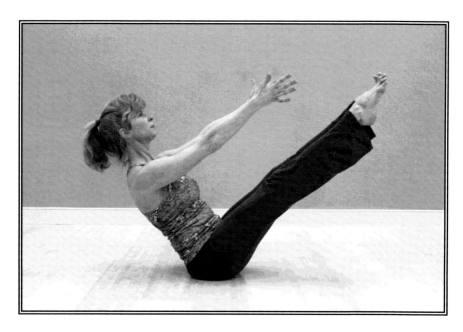

HOLD FOR 5 BREATHS

Transition: Inhale bending the knees into the chest and extending through the spine. Cross the ankles. Place hands by hips and lift the body off the ground for one breath. Repeat **Boat** pose and transition 3 times. Rock and roll forward and backward, massaging the spine. Go through half a vinyasa stopping in **Downward Facing Dog** to prepare for our next pose.

Hip-Opening Poses

Our whole life story is stored in the hips. We enter this world open, untainted and free. We are flexible and agile. As we move through life, our participation, injuries, work and emotional experiences become stored in our bodies, especially our hips. This area tightens and muscles contract. Over time, the body tissues shorten and limit mobility. This restriction in turn impacts joint range of motion and appropriate blood flow to important ligaments and tendons. Athletes may be particularly sensitive to hip-opening poses due to their prior conditioning. Approach these asanas with great care, gentleness and receptivity. Opening the hip areas of the body can be physically, mentally and emotionally revealing. If pain is encountered, slowly transition out of the pose. However, reasonable discomfort is expected and this is where growth lies. We learn in life by confronting that which presents a struggle with grace, humility and integrity.

The hips and supporting muscles are like the axis of the body. Upper and lower body movement is contingent upon strength and flexibility in this area. The hip-opening poses are designed to stimulate mobility and relieve tension. These postures will strengthen and stretch critical muscles that are instrumentally linked to overall health and well-being. They will address tightness and imbalance in our primary supporting muscles of the leg, lower back, and hip areas including the iliacus, psoas and piriformis.

At this point in our practice, our bodies are ready to let go. The muscles are warm. The mind and ego have taken a back seat. And, the axis of our being is available for awakening. As the practice moves into the hip-opening asanas, a keen awareness of breath and gaze will induce relaxation. Intentionally focus on the Ujjayi pranayama as we explore three poses and experience the physical, mental and emotional release.

Pose 31: Half Pigeon Pose
(Adho Mukha Eka Pada Rajakapotasana)

From **Downward facing dog** position, inhale extending the right leg upward. Exhale and step the right foot forward between the hands. Walk the right foot over toward the left corner of the mat. Bend the right leg at a 90-degree angle and flex the foot. With knee to ankle alignment parallel to the front edge, lower right leg to rest on the mat. Extend the back leg with the knee down, inner thigh rotating up. Toes and top of foot are pressing into the floor. Inhale and exhale while gently extending the upper body forward. Relax through the upper body and sink into this stress-relieving pose. This position will most likely be somewhat uncomfortable. Our bodies carry the majority of stress in our hip region. Breathe through the discomfort. Modification: move the right heel in closer to the pubis narrowing the degree of bend from the knee. Drishti: spot on the floor or tip of the nose.

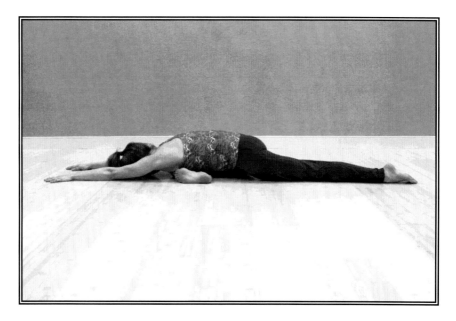

HOLD FOR 10 BREATHS

Transition: Inhale and slowly walk the hands toward the hips extending through the spine. Bring torso upright. Exhale rolling onto the right buttocks and fold the left leg at a 90 degree angle underneath the right setting up for our next pose, **Double Pigeon**.

Pose 32: Double Pigeon Pose
(Dwapada Rajakapotasana)

Stack the shins on top of each other with both legs at 90-degree angles. Allow the right ankle to dangle past the left knee/thigh. Lift the buttocks slightly up and backward. Move the flesh of the buttocks away, in order to rest on the sitting bones. Actively flex the feet. Inhale extending through the spine and lifting up. Exhale, hinging and folding forward from the hips. Drishti: spot on the floor or tip of the nose

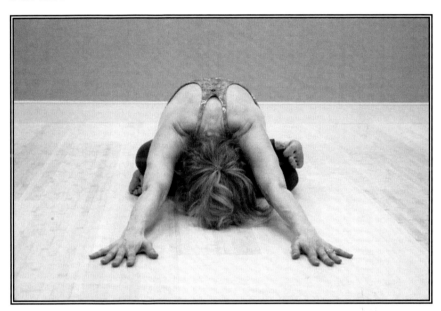

HOLD FOR 10 BREATHS

Transition: Inhale and slowly return to a seated upright position. Exhale and tighten the leg position inward toward the body. Bring the right knee facing forward. Left knee stacked directly beneath the right. Heels are parted just enough to allow sitting bones to rest between.

73

Pose 33: Cow Face Pose (Gomukhasana)

Seated between feet, knees are stacked. The toes point back. Sitting bones are resting between the feet. Inhale and bring left elbow upward, bicep by ear, fingertips reaching down between the shoulder blades. Exhale and bend the right arm up and behind the body, fingertips reaching upward between shoulder blades. Bind fingers together. Inhale pressing the base of the skull gently into the left forearm. Exhale folding forward from the hips. Extend through the spine and allow the base of the throat to move over top of the knees. Drishti: spot on the floor or tip of the nose.

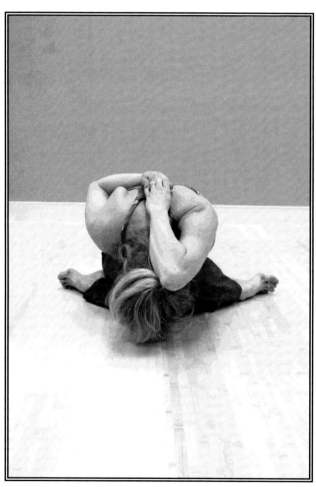

HOLD FOR 5 BREATHS

Transition: Inhale slowly returning to a seated upright position. Exhale and unravel the legs. Hug the knees to the chest. Rock and roll forward and backward, massaging the spine. Go through half a vinyasa stopping in **Downward Facing Dog.** Repeat poses 31 through 33 on the left side. Come to a seated position with both legs extended out in front of the body. Torso upright in preparation for **Head to Knee** pose.

Closing Series

The **Closing Series** can encompass a plethora of poses. This book will explore six fundamental and restorative asanas. In **One-Yoga**, these are sitting, lying, inverted and resting asanas. They include neutral, forward-bending, and twisting movements. The timing and placement of the poses at the end of the class is structured to:

- increase flexibility,
- improve joint range of motion,
- aid the functions of the digestive system,
- stimulate blood flow throughout the endocrine system
- promote stillness
- quiet the mind, and
- foster meditative serenity.

Some poses promote blood flow to the head, neck, throat and face. These postures assist the functions of the endocrine glands. Other postures support the health of the digestive system. Most closing-series forward bends are designed to induce a state of calm and well-being.

These asanas are the fruit of our labor. The entire practice leads up to this point. The class ends with our fifth component—**Relaxation** and **Meditation (Dhyana)**. Meditation is very personal, and there are many aspects of meditating that are common to all people. Although techniques for meditation and guided relaxation can vary, the general purpose is to stop the endless chatter of the mind and find a sense of stillness. It is in this stillness that we allow our hearts to be exposed and our spirits to connect.

> The Merriam-Webster's Dictionary definition of **Meditation** is: *the act or process of meditating; to engage in mental exercise (as concentration on one's breathing or repetition of a mantra) for the purpose of reaching a heightened level of spiritual awareness.*

First, let me say, I am not an expert on the practice of meditation. I have only learned from experience what works for me. As you approach these concluding poses, bring your awareness to the five senses. Smell, taste and see. Listen with the ears of the non-seeing. Hear the noises in the room, outside and within your body. Feel every morsel of your being as it connects to the earth. When a thought enters your mind, allow it to pass through without judgment. You are suspended and supported by the vibrations of the universe. You don't need to search for the divine, for it resides within. Go with the flow and just be.

Pose 34: Head to Knee Pose (Janu Sirsasana)

Bend the left knee, opening the hip. Bring the base of the left foot in to rest on the right inner thigh, allowing the knee to fold open. Dynamically activate the right quadriceps, flex the foot, and spread the toes. Inhale and lift the arms overhead. When exhaling, fold forward, extending over the right leg. Hinge at the hips and reach through the crown of the head. Take hold of the right foot with both hands and allow the chin and forehead to move toward the knee. If flexibility allows, drape the torso over the extended leg. Modification: Place both hands on either side of the right leg or take hold of the shin, flattening through the back. Inhale and exhale deeply. Permit the spine to elongate and create space. Drishti: Knee or big toe.

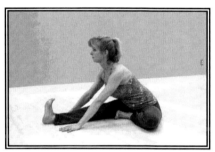 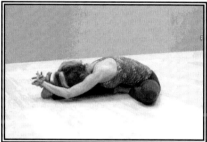

HOLD FOR 5 BREATHS

Transition: Inhale, reaching out and upward returning to a seated upright position. Exhale and cross the left foot over the right leg in preparation for **Seated Twist** pose.

Pose 35: Seated Twist Pose (Marichyasana)

While there are a number of variations to this pose, we will explore a basic cross-legged seated twist.

Right leg is extended. Left knee bent facing upward. Root down through the mound under the left big toe to ground the body and leverage the spinal twist. Inhale and raise both arms overhead. Exhale and begin to twist left from the belly button. Place the right bicep on the outside of the left thigh or wrap the right arm around the left leg. Place the left hand on the floor at the midline of the body near the buttocks. Inhale and extend through the crown of the head and elongating through the spine. Exhale and twist deeper. Drishti: Over the shoulder.

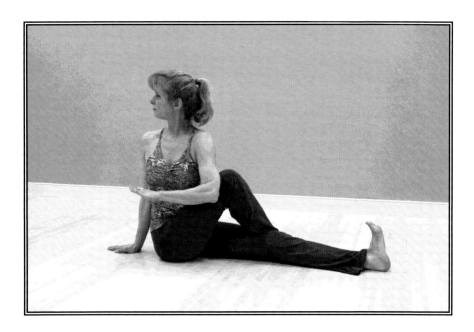

HOLD FOR 5 BREATHS

Transition: Inhale and release head, neck, shoulders and torso to face front. Exhale and bring both legs extended out in front. Repeat poses 34, 35 and transition on the other side.

Pose 36: Seated Forward Bend (Paschimottanasana)

Start with both legs extended out in front of the body. Torso is upright. Body and legs form a 90-degree angle. Move flesh away from sitting bones to encourage an erect long spine. Legs are together. Feet are flexed, toes spread apart. Inhale and lift the arms directly overhead shoulder distance width. Exhale and fold forward, hinging at the hips. Lead with the heart. If flexibility allows, extend the entire torso over the legs, placing the forehead on the knees/shins. Breathe. Modification: Place the hands on either side of the legs or on the shins and extend through the spine. Allow the breath to deepen this wonderful hamstring and lumbar stretch. Drishti: Big toes, knees or tip of the nose.

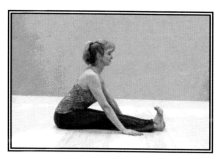 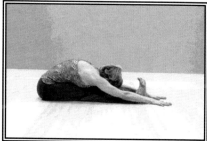

HOLD FOR 5 BREATHS

Transition: Inhale and come out of the pose the same way you entered it. Exhale softening the knees and rolling back supine one vertebra at a time.

Pose 37: Supine Spinal Twist
(Urdhva Jathara Parivartanasana)

From a reclined position, inhale and lift the right knee, hugging the knee to the chest. Place your arms out to the sides shoulder height with palms down or use the left hand to carry the right knee across the body. Exhale and engage through the abdominals, drawing the bellybutton toward the spine. Strive to keep both shoulders down. Relax the neck. Drishti: Gaze over the right shoulder.

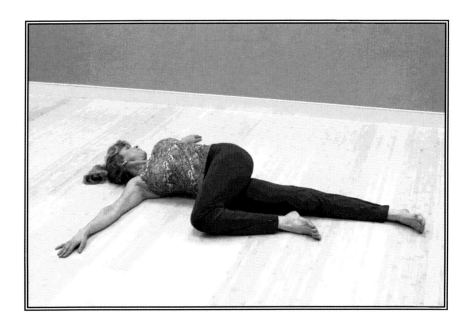

HOLD FOR 5 BREATHS

Transition: Inhale, engaging through the core and bring the knees into the chest. Exhale and switch sides with resting gaze over the left shoulder. Repeat transition. Slowly lower and extend both legs preparing for **Savasana**.

Pose 38: Corpse Pose (Savasana)

Lay on your back. Arms are extended about 6 inches to either side of the hips. Palms face up. Gently slide the shoulder blades down the spine moving away from the ears. Feet are splayed open about hip distance width, coming to rest in their natural position. Completely let go. Relax through the face and the throat. Let your heart soften and release any breath control. Allow your muscles to fall into the earth. And rest – just rest. Be still and be.

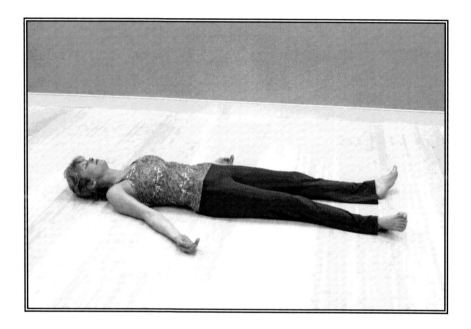

STAY IN SAVASANA FOR AS LONG AS NEEDED

When practicing **Savasana**, let go. Detach from conscious thought. As you tune into the sensations of your body, relinquish all control and enjoy the peace.

Transition: Bring awareness back to the body. Start moving the fingers and hands, toes and feet. Consciously begin to breathe. Slowly and lovingly bend one knee and then the other. Allow the knees to fall over to the right side of the body into a fetal position.

Pose 39: Infant / Fetal Pose (Dimbhasana)

The fetal or infant pose is that of a new born child. Knees are drawn in toward the abdomen. Arms bent in close to the body. Keep your eyes closed and enjoy this nurturing position.

HOLD FOR 2 – 5 BREATHS OR LONGER IF NEEDED

Transition: Using the hands, press into the earth and come to a seated cross-legged position. Bring your hands in heart center, hands in prayer position. Inhale and lift hands to the forehead (the third-eye center). Exhale and fold forward. Namaste'.

Conclusion

At the conclusion of the practice, you may be reflective, emotional and even blissful. It's my experience that yoga practice helps us to learn or re-learn how to love ourselves. And, in loving ourselves right here and right now – the judgment and self-criticism melts away. As judgment leaves, it is replaced by acceptance, awareness, life of the present moment and joy. We become better people.

This profound practice changes our perspective on everything by bringing focus, attention and clarity to our conscious. It physically, mentally, and emotionally strips away the outer shell we have encrusted ourselves in, and opens the way for our being to flourish.

There is so much more to learn and experience. Being a student is a lifelong experience. My recommendation for everyone is to continue to practice regularly. It is the consistency of practice that guides self-discovery and self-realization.

One-Yoga's Power Flow Yoga was born out of requests from my students and fellow practioners who wanted to learn a particular style of yoga. It evolved over my lifetime. It is based on my training, self-development and life experiences using a straightforward, common-sense approach to the spiritual and physical practice of yoga.

Teaching yoga is one of the greatest gifts I have received. It is an act of giving without expecting anything in return. And when done so fully, students share their light. That is the greatest reward. In guiding and helping students to find their inner peace, I have been given the gift of love, connection and purpose. Thank you for being present.

Blessings,

Susan L. Smith

Bibliography & Resources

Baptiste, Baron. 2002. *Journey Into Power.* New York, NY.

Baptiste, Baron. 2004. *40 Days to Personal Revolution.* New York, NY.

Beattie, Melody. 1996. *Journey to the Heart.* New York, NY.

Belling, Noa. 2001. *The Yoga Handbook.* New Holland Publishers, U.K.

Burgin, Timothy. 2006. *Yoga Basics, Focusing on a Drishti.* Asheville, N.C. Available at: http://www.yogabasics.com.

Coulter, David H. 2001. *Anatomy of Hatha Yoga.* Honesdale, PA.

Devereux, Godfrey. 1998. *Dynamic Yoga.* Hammersmith, London.

Frawley, Dr. David. 1999. *Yoga & Ayurveda Self Healing and Self-Realization.* Twin Lakes, Wisconsin.

Gaspar, Lori. 2003. *The Many Nuances of Vinyasa.* Chicago, IL. Available at: http://www.yogachicago.com.

Iyengar, B.K.S. 1993. *Light on the Yoga Sutras of Pantanjali.* Hammersmith, London. Available at: www.bksiyengar.com.

Merriam-Webster Online Dictionary. 2005. *Definition of Meditation and Meditating.* Springfield, MA. http://www.m-w.com (accessed March 2007).

Ramacharaka, Yogi. 1903. *Hindu-Yogi, Science of Breath.* Ludgate Hill, London. Available at: http://www.arfalpha.com.

Swenson, David. 1999. *Ashtanga Yoga, The Practice Manual.* Austin, TX.

Wikipedia Encyclopedia. 2002. *Definition of Asana.* Boston, MA. www.wikipedia.org (accessed March 2007).